"Nice guys DO finish first! / ight into how Cornell McBride gu kets and new directions yet never once gave up the family-oriented qualities that made him successful. The book is final proof that the old American formula for business success—intimacy, a reliance on employees, the free-flow of ideas, and innovation—is still the best way to be #1."

—Lafayette Jones, President and Chief Executive Officer of *Segmented Marketing Services* and *Urban Call Publishing*

"One of the classiest, savviest and most suave businessmen you'll ever meet...Cornell McBride's philosophy is simple: Putting people first—and that includes your employees—means bigger profits. There are very few executives who so enjoy their lives and careers as much as Cornell. I only wish he could be cloned and placed on the board of every Fortune 500 company."

—Bob Johnson, Founder and Chairman, *BET/Black Entertainment Television*

"The history of the evolution of the African-American hair-care business in this country would not be complete without this riveting rags-to-riches story of a young Black boy growing up in the rural south who went on to found one of the most successful Black-owned businesses in the country today. Walk with Cornell McBride, Sr., as he takes us on his very personal journey from those modest beginnings to running a wildly successful business that nearly shattered his life to his 'getting back on his feet' and starting over. Cornell McBride, Sr., has written a brilliant, illuminating book that is an essential read for anyone who wants to truly understand Black America, Black Business and Black History—and for anyone who just wants to read a wonderfully inspiring book!"

—Bonnie L. Krueger, Publishing, Editorial Services Director, *Sophisticate's Black Hair Magazine*

"*A Cut Above* is a remarkable memoir: frank, refreshing, fascinating, and charming. This book reveals the author's secrets for success in both business and in life. It really hits the mark by seamlessly blending the practical with the inspirational. Not many people have endured what McBride has been through and still come out on top. His story is remarkable. This book is simply superb!"

—Honorable Andrew Young Chairman, *GoodWorks International*, Atlanta, Georgia, Former Mayor of Atlanta, Civil Rights Activist, Former U.S. Ambassador to the United Nations

"My friend and fellow pharmacist Cornell McBride has always had his eye on the American dream. From the very first time I met him over 25 years ago, when *Sally Beauty Supply* began distributing Sta Sof Fro products, I could tell from his determination, entrepreneurial spirit and 'can do' attitude that he would indeed reach his goals. This book is his fast-moving story of his company's successes and failures and his unshakable will to always come out on top."

—Michael H. Renzulli, R.Ph, Chairman,
Sally Beauty Company

"Cornell McBride has been a business associate and personal friend for over 20 years. He is one of the brightest and classiest entrepreneurs in our business. His passion for people, his personal warmth, great sense of humor and hands-on involvement make him a role model for nice guys trying to succeed in a tough business environment. This book is an honest account of Cornell's personal life, his career and the sound advice and counsel he so willingly shares with young people motivated to achieve. Simply said, it's a great read and highly entertaining."

—Jay Forbes, VP Customer Development,
Drug Store News

"He distills a lifetime of winning strategies and formulas for success. It is not lost that the foundation gained from his pharmacy education facilitated the selection of ingredients and the effective blending into ingenious hair care products. And, that basic principles learned in pharmacy administration courses guided business development and under-girded strategies. Pharmacists and pharmacy students will find guidance for their careers and studies in this life story."

—Johnnie L. Early, II, Ph.D, R.Ph, Dean and Professor,
The University of Toledo College of Pharmacy

"Inspiring, motivational, emotional, and exciting! Cornell McBride embodies the American Dream and this is the story of one man's rise and fall—and how he rose again. Anyone who wants success in business and in life ought to read this book. This isn't simply a 'how-to' manual, it's a lesson by example. Mr. McBride shows us the very essence of perseverance, commitment, discipline, and entrepreneurial spirit."

—Angela Marcano, author of *African American Heiress*

To: all the best. Cornell McBride S

A Cut Above

*How the Man Who Gave the World
the Afro Made $$ Millions!*

Cornell McBride

MRL Publishing

A Cut Above: How the Man Who Gave the World the Afro Made $$ Millions!
Copyright © 2006 Cornell McBride
MRL Publishing

For more information on this title, please contact:
MRL Publishing
P.O. Box 1615 Lithonia, Georgia 30058
Lameisha Estelle (770) 593-7221
lameishaestelle@mcbrideresearchlabs.com

Cover Photo by Ernest Washington at www.edupphoto.com

Book design by Arbor Books
www.arborbooks.com

Printed in Canada

ISBN: 0-9768595-0-5 —softcover

LCCN: 2005926271

Affectionately dedicated to my parents, Eddie Will and Thelma McBride–who inspired me with their dedication to family and simple, but profound view of life. To my wife, Harriet, who believed in me and supported my desire to be an entrepreneur. To my children Sheila (in loving memory), Sholanda, Cornell Jr. and Andre, a beautiful bunch. To all the employees of M&M Products whose tireless effort contributed to the company's success. To my friend Beverly Kieveman Copen who encouraged me to write this book.

Acknowledgements

There are countless people to thank and acknowledge for their inspiration, their help and support—my Air Force buddies, wonderful college mentors, business associates and loyal friends, my parents and siblings. The list is long, that's for sure. But I give special mention to Therman McKenzie, my partner; Jackie Archer of NAACP, Lloyd Archer, Air Force Master Sergeant Rudy Holmes, Annie Washington, from Mercer School of Pharmacy. And I owe a debt of gratitude to Katie and Ralph, who helped and encouraged me during the early years. Larry Leichman, The Floating Gallery for managing this book and keeping me on track. Mia Claudia Wood, for her assistance in writing this book.

Contents

Preface

I come from very humble beginnings. I am the fifth child in a family of eight children. When I was growing up, I remember having dreams of a better life, a strong desire to do right and a will to succeed. My parents instilled in me a strong moral foundation and the strong will to succeed springs from my own determination to fulfill a promise. These factors motivated me to become the person I am today.

When I was 10 years old, I promised my mother that I would build her a house. I didn't know exactly how I would do it, but that promise was always at the back of my mind. My childhood was difficult to say the least, but the mysterious yet nagging entrepreneurial spirit I had helped me to achieve difficult goals in a short period of time. The experience of growing up first as a poor child in the segregated South, then as a young man looking for opportunities at the height of the civil rights movement forced me to forge my own way in a discriminatory society. That lesson has proven to be one of the most important ingredients in the recipe for my business success.

To this day, I am so thankful for the values that my parents instilled in me and my siblings. They taught us that integrity was the most important sign of good character. It is that lesson that keeps me honest and upright in everything I do. I try to exemplify these principles with the people who work with me, for me and with everyone I come into contact in my daily life.

An equally important ingredient to life and success in business is discipline. To me discipline is controlling yourself in every aspect of life—from getting up in the morning, to working hard, to never living beyond your means. Discipline is staying focused and not getting distracted by obstacles along the way. In doing so, the mind is free to be creative. Worrying about too many things hinders creativity.

I had been a witness to and the recipient of so many wrongdoings in my life that right along with discipline and integrity was my desire to always do the right thing. To me, doing the right thing is even closer to Godliness than cleanliness. I believe in taking care of my responsibilities, family comes first, and I believe it is important to make decisions that will ensure your family's security, even if that means taking risks. To take a risk, you must have a good idea that what you're doing has a good chance of succeeding, and you should not be swayed by doubt or hardships.

My era may have been different from today's but the lessons I learned, and the values I've lived by, are as relevant today as they were when I was coming up. Though many more opportunities are available today than when I was a child and young man, it is still true that anyone who wants to make their mark in life has to find and develop the opportunities that do come along—and even better, to make one's own opportunities.

This story is about my life, but it's also about anyone who has dreams of making life better than it is right now. If my life story inspires people to change their lives, that's because the values that have driven me throughout my life exist today—and they are here for everyone. Society sometimes forgets about the values like hard work, honesty, and discipline, but they're still here, and they're just as good as they were when God placed us on this earth.

I found that in owning a business you want to create an environment that encourages people to be their best, to fulfill their capacities, and maybe even surprise themselves with what they can accomplish. Starting and growing not one, but two, successful Afro-American hair-care product companies, has taught me what works and what does not in this highly competitive business.

When my college friend Therman McKenzie and I started M&M Products Company in Georgia in the early 1970s, we had no idea how successful we would become. I was co-owner of one of the most successful black-owned companies in America, and a millionaire by the time I was 35. My success was completely unexpected. After all, the sort of success I achieved surpassed any notion I had of what success would look like. Still, I had worked hard, and was constantly thinking about how I could improve the business. The sky was the limit, or so I thought

Though we surpassed our expectations for success, we also surpassed our expectations for failure. When

M&M was finally sold, it was one of the saddest times of my life. But I found that failure is not a life sentence, so long as you have solid values for living to fall back on. The lifelong lessons learned on Mom's tables were a big help at those trying times. The values of hard work, discipline, honesty and integrity have provided the foundation for success—and a net of security when things failed.

For years, people have wanted to know the story of M&M's rise and subsequent deterioration. I decided that now is the time to tell that story, and in telling it, I also tell the story of my life.

—*Cornell McBride*

Chapter 1: Sugar Hill

"I'm going to build you a house some day," I declared to my mother. She paused at the kitchen sink and turned her sweet face toward me. "That's a promise," I continued. Standing before her, my 10-year-old frame already mirrored hers—long, slender body and richly dark complexion. She smiled at me warmly. "Yes, it's a promise. I'm saving my money," I said as proof of my intention.

Indeed, I was saving. Every day of that year, in 1953, I put in at least a penny into a tin Carnation milk can that I kept hidden from my siblings. I stashed it under my bed, or behind a dresser, anywhere I felt it would be safe from sticky fingers. And I never let anyone see me. I finally broke into the can for something I wanted, but the promise had been made, and I was determined to keep it. After all, I had a mother who inspired such devotion.

Every day after school, or after a long humid summer day of play, Mom was cooking something up in the kitchen of our mill house at the Sugar Refinery Quarters—better known to us as Sugar Hill. She always made sure we had something good to eat.

What she managed to do for ten people on just a few dollars a week—not just buy food but pay the household bills and outfit all us kids with school supplies and such—was the closest thing to a miracle I have ever experienced.

There were ten of us: my parents, Thelma and Eddie Will McBride, and eight kids. Two years separated each of us. Earl, the eldest, was eight years older than I. Next was Willie, then Rose Lee, whom we called Rose. After her was Bernice, who was just ahead of me; I was fifth and was followed by Garfield. He and I were pretty much inseparable throughout childhood. The last two McBride kids were Eddie and Richard.

Our mother took care of every last one of us with tender love and devotion. Once a week she would shop for groceries. Most often, my father would take her to the store. There were times, however, that he was not available, and those occasions stick out in my memory to this day. When she did not have a ride to the store, she would walk, because ride or no ride, mother was going to make sure you ate. I can still see her carrying those bags toward our house, stopping every few feet or so along the dusty road to set them down and rest. The first time I saw her pause like that, I ran out to help her the rest of the way home. At that moment, I decided that I would take care of her.

The Saturday after I made my announcement to my mom, the whole family was in the car on our way home from downtown Savannah after a day's shopping. I was in the back seat, playing and carrying on with my brothers and sisters, when I overheard my mom and dad talking up front.

"You know what, Eddie Will?" my mother asked. She always called my father "Eddie Will."

"Say, Old Lady," he replied. Old Lady was his nickname for my mother, and he spoke the words with such deep affection.

"Cornell's going to build us a house."

My dad looked over at my mom and chuckled. "Oh, he is?"

"That's right. And he's even saving his money," she answered with a smile.

I didn't say anything, but I thought, "Yes, I am." What I'd told my mother was no idle promise. I intended not just to keep it, but to live up to it as fast as I could. That promise became my guiding light to become successful in life, and I always remembered it.

My father was a laborer, and he was built for it. Almost six feet tall, with limbs as thick as barrels, he weighed about 230 pounds. He had a decent job with the Sugary Refinery Corporation mill where they made Dixie Crystal Sugar, the brand in most American women's kitchens in those times. Those were good days—hard, but still good for a black family living in the segregated South, since we lived according to the limited means a black family could achieve in a world where blacks were given few options. In those days, black people did not make a lot of money, about half of what whites made. Still, our house was nice in comparison with other housing for blacks in Georgia and the rest of the South.

Sugar Hill consisted of a couple of rows of stand-alone, clapboard box houses on either side of the train tracks, just about five miles outside of downtown

Savannah—whites on one side and blacks on the other. Everyone who lived there worked at the refinery. It was a nice enough place to grow up in. The mill houses, though small, had indoor plumbing, which was a rarity, so we had running water and a bathroom inside. The housing was cheap, too, and even if you didn't make a lot working at the refinery, you still had a nice house to go home to in a safe neighborhood.

Unlike many young black children in America in the 1940s and 1950s, I grew up with the advantages of parents who stuck to that American work ethic despite the obstacles, and I grew up largely in the safety of a small but stable community. My parents had created a life that, for them, was successful.

They came up in Georgia during the depression, where education was not a part of black life, let alone opportunities to make enough money to scrape together a life. My father was born in 1913, and my mom six years later, and later the depression made an already hard life even harder. As a result, neither one of my parents were able to finish elementary school. Not being able to read or write was the norm in those days. Still, my parents were so worldly-wise and full of experience that I did not know they could not read or write beyond their own names until I was in the third grade.

Looking back, I know my parents struggled, but they created an environment that made us feel loved and secure. It was my parents who instilled in us the virtues of hard work, honesty and fairness that I rely on to this very day. Both of my parents taught us every day about what sort of people they expected us to become.

In our community, it was expected that people worked hard at the mill. One generation after another grew up and went to work for the Refinery Corporation. That is just what I thought I would do—grow up, get married and work at the sugar refinery.

Still something inside me drove me on from the beginning in a way that would take me far beyond the fence of my neighborhood. Of course I did not know it then. Whatever it was that urged me on, even before I made my promise, I knew early on that my life would change, and in changing, I would help others in my family. I had appointed myself the person who would help my family because I thought that if I didn't become successful, no one would.

The older McBride children began dropping out of school to work at the mill or get married themselves when they were about 17. Earl, Willie, Rose and Bernice had all left high school before graduating. It was common for 16- and 17-year-olds in and around our neighborhood to work in the mill.

I knew that becoming a success and building my mother a house meant I needed money. Learning how to earn the money I would one day use to care for my parents and my own family began early in my life. There was the example of money management my mother set at home and through her housecleaning work, and there was my father's example as head of our household and the disciplinarian. As the household disciplinarian, he was the one we feared if we got caught doing something wrong, and that structure kept us on the straight and narrow for the most part.

Most kids in my neighborhood could go into

Savannah on a Saturday to see a matinee movie because their parents would give them the 50 cents for the cost of the movie. But I learned quickly not to ask my dad for the money.

"Daddy," I said one Saturday morning. I couldn't have been more than 10 or 12. "A bunch a kids are goin' down to the theater. I want to go, too."

He looked down at me and said, "You do? Well, then I suppose you're going to have to figure out pretty fast how to get the money for that ticket."

It didn't take me long to realize that if I wanted to go to a matinee on Saturday, I had to start planning my jobs on Monday in order to earn enough money for the movie. I did odd jobs for my neighbors—pretty much whatever job I needed to do in order to earn my 50 cents was what I did. Later, I began creating businesses like mowing lawns and gathering scrap iron and copper with my friends from the refinery dump every day after school. After we collected enough, we would take to the junkyard to sell. Pretty soon I was often earning enough money not only to go to an occasional Saturday movie, but also to buy my own school supplies and pay for my own school lunch. My mom had always given me a quarter every day, but I knew she needed it, so I started refusing to take it, and instead tried to pay on my own.

I was pretty industrious, too. Along with odd jobs I picked up around my neighborhood, I kept coming up with some idea or other to make money. When I was about 10 years old, I got together $5 and planned to buy a hog from Abram Bowens. Mr. Abram was the school bus driver, but like most folks, he had a sideline.

His was raising hogs. I thought I could become a hog farmer, too. I got a pen fixed up in the backyard.

My brother Willie, who watched me work, offered to help. "If you give me your $5, I could get you that pig."

"Really?" I said, wiping dirt and sweat from my forehead. I had worked hard in the sweltering summer sun to prepare a pen, but there was still much to do, and having Willie pick up my pig would save me time. "Okay." I dug into my trouser pocket and pulled out five crumpled dollar bills.

I got everything set up and then waited. And waited. But there was no Willie. I went inside. "Momma, have you seen Willie?"

She was at the kitchen counter cutting vegetables. "No, I haven't seen him all day. But he'd better be back for dinner."

"He's supposed to get my pig from Mr. Abrams," I said, feeling uneasy.

Eventually, Willie came back but without my pig. He sauntered into the kitchen, as nonchalant as can be. "Willie," I demanded. "Where's my pig?"

"What pig?"

"What pig!" I was irate. "You have got to be kidding. *My* pig. The one you were supposed to get from Mr. Abram."

"Oh, I don't have it," he said casually, as if that explained everything.

"How can you not have it? I gave you the mo—" suddenly I stopped. "My money. Where's my money? Give me my $5 back!"

He picked up a stalk of celery off the counter and took a bite. "I don't have it."

I was dumbfounded. "You don't have it," I repeated.

"Nope."

"But it's *my* money. How can you not have my money?"

"I just don't."

The angrier I got, the more he seemed to melt into slow motion. He just sort of shrugged off every question and every demand.

Finally, I turned to our mother, who had been quietly working at the counter. "Momma, he stole my money. Make him give it back!"

Without turning around, she said, "Willie, why don't you give that boy his money?" She was a mild-mannered woman of few words, but the ones she spoke she intended to have an impact. If they did not, she was not the sort of person to waste her time pushing. On those rare occasions she did get upset, you'd better watch out, but apparently, this was not one of them.

"But I don't have it," was all he said. And that was that. I never did get my $5 back, and Willie never would tell me what he did with it. I vowed after that always to keep track of every penny that I had.

Needless to say, I was known in the family as the one who had the money. I was the businessman, and I guess Willie thought it wasn't anything at all for me to spare that money. Still, I stayed optimistic. I soon got over the loss of my $5, but it was a long time before I forgave my brother Willie.

Another time, a few years later when we moved out of Sugar Hill, I tried to become a turkey farmer. Up the street from the dilapidated old house on Highway 17 was a chicken and turkey farm. Somehow I managed to buy a young female turkey, and brought it home with plans of selling its eggs and raising more turkeys. But day after day, and then week after week, that turkey did nothing but walk around, eat and sleep. Every day I fed her, cleaned out her coop, and looked for the jewel that I was sure she'd make for me. But despite all my efforts, she did not lay even one egg. One morning as I made my way into the house, long-faced after experiencing yet another empty nest, my mother wiped her hands on her apron and turned to me with that warm smile.

"Cornell, you know you tried hard. Sometimes things just don't quite go the way you plan, but you keep trying."

I nodded my head dejectedly.

"You know what?"

I shrugged. "What?"

"I bet we can still find a use for that turkey."

I looked up at her hopefully. We did find a use for it, and that turkey did not taste half bad.

Chapter 2: A Child of Segregation

I did not know anything different from the life I was born into, and that was a life of segregation. At the same time, I did not know from the beginning what it was. I did not realize how significant were those train tracks that separated the white kids from us. There were 37 homes on each side, and though we would see the white kids every day, there wasn't much interaction. There were times, though, when we kids just wanted to play more than we wanted to follow the unwritten rules separating us in our own backyards, and we would get together to make up an informal ball game. Play had nothing to do with color, and we knew that. Besides, there wasn't much else to do besides playing ball or hunting in the woods for birds, and it was natural for all the kids to want to get together to have some fun.

But then it wouldn't be long before somebody went and told Joe Morgan, the refinery's hired security. We called him "the police" even though we knew he wasn't, because he still had just about that much authority over us. Whenever all the Sugar Hill kids got together he'd come around and break it up, sometimes right in the middle of a really good game.

"Go on! Get on home," he would holler, and we would scatter, separating onto either side of the tracks. Then, until the next time we summoned the courage to cross again to each other, we would pretty much stick to our own sides.

In those days it was simply expected that everyone who lived in Sugar Hill kept to the rules. If you didn't, you lose jobs and that also meant losing a good home. But in our family, that did not translate to lying down. Our parents taught us kids never to pick a fight, but not to back down if someone picked one with you. Avoiding a fight did not mean you were a coward. It meant that fighting should always be a last resort.

I did not accept the dehumanization of segregation as having the power to dehumanize *me*. There was no sense of inferiority or submissiveness to the long-standing culture bred by segregation. No one in my family ever said that they couldn't do something, or that there was no point in trying because it wouldn't matter, anyway. In fact, I don't believe those thoughts were even entertained in private, let alone uttered in family conversations. My parents may not have had much formal education, but they were proud people and lived their lives with dignity.

But even though strong, self-respecting parents raised me, and even though I did not submit to the oppression of segregation, I was confused about what segregation meant. For a brief period, when I was somewhere around age 8 or 9, I did think that the situation of black people had to be our own fault. Why else would something so awful as segregation, and the limited opportunities that are some of its consequences, exist if we didn't somehow bring them about ourselves? I thought this mainly because I was stymied in my own early attempts to succeed in a world that was both black and white. My first experience with the social organization based on the color dichotomy was when I played America's favorite pastime, baseball.

I loved playing baseball as a kid. At a young age I was already long-limbed and slender and seemed to be built well for playing ball. We would organize pick-up games, and I dreamt of spending my days on a baseball diamond. There was no organized team in our neighborhood, but the white kids had a nice field, neat uniforms, their own team, and they played every Saturday to cheering crowds. I thought that if I played with my friends, and I also played with the white team, that would mean I'd get to play twice as much, and this was just what I wanted. So I tried to join the local white league team. One afternoon I presented myself at practice, mitt and all, ready to play.

"Hey, Cornell," the coach said as I trotted up to the field. "What are you doin' here, son?"

"Coach, I want to play. I want to be on the team."

It was hot out, and the coach squinted through beads of sweat. "You what?" he asked, as if he hadn't heard me right.

"Wanna play. I want to play."

"Well, now, don't you boys already fix some games on your own?"

"Sure, but—"

"Cornell, that's where you need to play. This team here is for these boys. You all don't play together. You know that, right?" He'd asked me the question, more rhetorical than anything else, in something amounting to disbelief.

The boys had stopped playing, and slowly moved over to where the coach and I stood. They knew something was up. But they also knew not to cross their coach.

"I know it, Coach, but it's not fair. It's not right we can't all play together. It's just a game." I didn't mean it in any moral sense, it just seemed unnatural to me, and entirely unnecessary to keep separate games—especially when I knew you could have one fine team if all the good kids from both sides got to play together. What mattered to me was being on a good team, a winning team, not a black or a white one. And this team, that happened to be white, was a winning one. It couldn't have been simpler in my young mind.

The coach, who was as nice a white man as many other nice white men in our community, sighed deeply. "I know it's hard to understand, but one day you will. I'm sorry, Cornell, I truly am." With an edge in his voice he sent the other boys back to their practice, and then turned back to me. "You want to maybe shag some balls? We could do that."

I nodded vigorously. "Yes!"

So, for a while I was allowed to practice a little pitching and field some balls. I truly believed that if I proved to be a good enough player, the coach would put me on the team. What mattered to me was that I was on that field and that I had a chance to earn a place on that baseball team. Hadn't I been taught that hard work and competence paid off?

"Coach?" I asked cautiously one day after weeks of practicing with the team.

"Uh-huh?" he answered absentmindedly as he gathered up equipment.

"I'm never going to play, am I?"

Suddenly, he stopped what he was doing, and turned around to face me. He looked frightened, almost, as if I had just caught him stealing. "Well, now, Cornell," he started. But then he just sort of trailed off. We stood there awkwardly for a moment. Finally, he said, "You know what I told you right off."

"Yes."

"I never promised anything."

"I know it. I just thought if I was good enough—"

"You *are* good enough," he interrupted. "Son, don't ever think you aren't good enough. I told you, it's not about you."

I'd been let down easy by the coach when he let me hang out with the team, but I was let down nonetheless. It was a peculiar sort of thing to have a white person such as the coach like me, yet feel compelled not to treat me the same as he would his own child just because of some rules set up long before he arrived. Didn't he know that if he and others didn't follow those rules, they wouldn't have any power at all? But as long as I hung around, all I'd ever get to do was practice a little for a game I'd never be allowed to play.

"You know what, Coach?" I asked, still standing before him.

"Say."

"It should be about me."

"You're right about that, Cornell. It should be."

I went home, confused and sad. But by the time I got home, I was angry. "What do *they* know?" I demanded, storming into the kitchen. I threw my hat and mitt on the table.

"What does who know?" my ever-present mother asked. "And pick up your things. You know you don't go throwing stuff around this house."

"Yes, ma'am," I responded dejectedly.

She wiped her hands on her apron and knelt down in front of me. "Now, who are we talking about?"

"I don't know who, that's the problem! But they won't let us play together, and the white kids always got better everything. Better mitts and bats. Better uniforms."

She swallowed hard, and put her hands on my shoulders. "Cornell, you are going to find that sometimes, life is not fair. But where there's a will, there's a way."

"What do you mean?"

"I mean, that no matter what obstacles people put before you, if you want something bad enough, you can find a way to get it or get something like it. Take this baseball team. White folks have got themselves some crazy ideas. Okay, fine. You can't change them. But there are other ways to get what you want. You just have to keep your eyes open for the opportunity." She kissed me on my forehead and got up. "Remember that. Keep your eyes open." Then she turned back toward the sink. "It's like I tell you when you have a fight with one of your friends. You know, if they do you wrong."

"I know, I have to feed them out of a long-handled spoon."

She nodded, washing some vegetables in the sink. "That's right. You be kind, but you keep your distance. Besides, you can see more from a distance."

"Like opportunities?"

"That's right. Like opportunities."

A couple of years later, the refinery built separate basketball courts and football and baseball fields for us kids to play on, each with our own. There was also a little league for black kids, and we got the white team's cast-off uniforms and equipment. All this made clear we were to remain separate in life, but it still struck me as unreasonable to prevent black and white kids from playing with each other just because people decided that was the way things should be.

Chapter 3: Leaving Sugar Hill

Once I started opening my eyes, I saw just how big the world really was. It began, in part, with reading the newspaper. My best friend, Willie Palmer, lived a few houses down from us. I started going over to his house in the morning because they had the paper delivered. I'd sit on the porch steps reading the sports page. Like almost every black person, I was an avid fan of the Brooklyn Dodgers because they were the first major league team to have black players. They had Jackie Robinson and Roy Campanella, and the fact that the Brooklyn Dodgers recognized their greatness signaled the open-mindedness of that team.

After a while, I began to look at other sections of the paper, too, and I learned quickly there was a lot happening in the world beyond the sports page. The early 1950s was a time of profound social and global change. Everything from the aftermath at home of the Second World War to the burgeoning Civil Rights movement, to the Korean War and increasing tensions that would lead to the Cold War. Reading the paper introduced me to politics, which became a lifelong passion of mine. The whole political process fascinated me. I knew the leaders of both political parties, not just in the state of Georgia, but nationally. I did not realize it at the time, but I was educating myself about how things worked and what the forces that drove society forward were. It was a new world outside of my own, and I knew I wanted to see it and be a part of it. I just had to start figuring out a way to get there. Though I did not leave Savannah until I graduated from high school, there was plenty going on to keep me occupied until then.

My father, "Chick" McBride was not the sort of man who bridled or buckled simply because the color of your skin in those days largely determined how you were treated and what opportunities you had. He did not go against the system of segregation itself, but if you crossed him, if you did him or his family wrong, he didn't care if you were black, white, or purple he was going to fight you.

But he was also not allowed to be a complete man in society. One incident was especially cruel. When I was still a small child, a white man from across the tracks wanted to borrow my dad's mule, but he did not want to pay him for it. My father kept the mule to work neighboring fields for extra money, and he also kept a garden in the backyard of our house.

Well, this man who demanded to borrow the mule just expected my father to kowtow to him. But that arrangement was not acceptable to my father, and he refused. Just days later, the mule was dead. My father was certain the man who'd wanted to borrow the mule had cruelly killed it. He confronted the white man, but with no proof, there was nothing he could do about it. This devastated him. He'd stood up to so much and won, but this affected him like nothing else. Soon enough, he was down at Gordon Road, hanging out and drinking white lightnin' instead of plowing the fields when he wasn't at the refinery. Not being able to effect change in his own life was abhorrent to him, and it had shaken him to his core.

Gordon Road was a neighborhood next to Refinery Quarters, comprised of a combination of liquor houses and regular, hardworking people's homes. A liquor house was someone's home. You could go there and buy their homemade beer or hard liquor—it was like a bar, except not an officially recognized business. In fact, liquor houses were not exactly legal.

The mill community had no liquor houses and had no room for folks who weren't working at the refinery. So, Gordon Road became an area where people who were down on their luck or looking for something to drink congregated in the midst of others just trying to work an honest day and pay their rent.

I know my father tried hard, and he was a dignified man, but when he drank it was apparent that he could not be counted on to take care of his responsibilities. He was a different person with alcohol in his blood, not the strong father I knew. I marveled that he could stay off alcohol, that he worked hard, and so forth, but I could not reconcile this man with the one who drank. And the longer he drank, the harder my mother had to work, and the more we kids had to contribute to help keep the house together.

His experience and its effect on him and the family did not prevent him, however, from continuing to instill in his own children the concept of taking responsibility for creating their own futures. Nor did it keep him from teaching us that we should always stand up for ourselves. I often thought that if he had followed the advice he gave to his children, my father could have been tremendous. As it was, my father was something of a contradiction to me. He was unquestionably the head of our household, and when he wasn't drinking, he was a level-headed, responsible man who dispensed wonderful advice and strong guidance. He was also a man who could walk away from alcohol just as easily as he imbibed, and later in life quit drinking altogether. Although he drank most weekends, he always got up the following Monday morning to go to work.

One typically sweltering summer day when I was about 1 3 years old, my friends and I, the group of kids everyone at school called the Sugar Hill Boys, were walking down to Route 17, the main highway near our neighborhood. A car sped by filled with a bunch of white boys. As they passed, they pelted us with handfuls of nails, laughing uproariously as the car faded into the distance. We yelled and cursed, but there was no way to catch them. Fortunately, no one in our group was hurt much, but we were mad—mad enough to know we had to seek revenge, and plan it so that it would be felt by each and every one of those kids in that car.

We got them back, and good, a short time later. One of the boys was delivering papers at Sugar Hill, and

Garfield and I hid out with buckets of rocks and waited for him across the tracks. He arrived just as the train was passing, so that they were caught between the train and us. At that moment, we leapt out of our hiding places and began throwing rocks at him. He got bruised up a bit, but was otherwise unhurt.

"I hear you beat up on some white boy," my father said to me shortly thereafter. Word had got out that a group of black boys had attacked a white boy, and the whole thing became a racial incident. "Do you know whose son that is?"

"No, sir. But," I protested, "they attacked us first."

My father ignored my comment. "He's one of the managers' boys. And you know what that means?"

"No," I replied tentatively.

"That means we're going to have to leave here."

"What! But that's not fair! They pelted us—"

"It's not about fair," my father interrupted.

I was devastated. The prospect of moving out of our house disturbed all of us. For months we lived in fear that we would have to pack up and find another place to live outside Sugar Hill. The only good thing was that my dad would not lose his job because of me. Finally, however, I think through my dad's persistence, one of the mill supervisors found out the whole story, nails and all. We were given a reprieve because one person understood the truth about what had happened. Eddie "Chick" McBride's family would not have to move after all.

However, within a year or so after the nails and rocks incident, we were finally forced to leave the comfortable and affordable Sugar Hill house—though it was through

no fault of my father's. There was an incident between
him and his foreman that resulted in our eviction. From
what I heard, this foreman had a habit of gathering up a
bunch of his men and taking them to South Carolina,
where he had some land, and then setting them to work
it without paying them one red penny. My father balked
at every aspect of this arrangement. He wasn't about to
leave his family and travel up to South Carolina, then
work some white man's property and not even get paid
for it. He still worked at the mill, but now had to travel
a ways to get to work everyday.

The new house at Five Mile Bend gave me my first
experience with outdoor bathrooms, and there was no
running water inside, either. When I walked through
the house I was so shocked that a person could live
this way I thought we must have just traveled back in
time to the 1800s. The house was made of brick and
not well insulated, so that it was always either too hot
or too cold, neither temperature very appealing in a
coastal environment like Savannah. I had to ride my
bike about four miles every day, too, if I wanted to see
my friends at Sugar Hill.

We stayed in that house just about two years before
we moved again when I was about 15 years old. Though
I do not recall the reasons why we moved, I was happy
enough about the decision—until I saw the new place.

We moved into a creaky, drafty, dilapidated old
house on Highway 17. Compared with the mill house,
this one felt like a shack. There was no indoor plumbing in this place either, and worst of all, it felt like we
were in the middle of the sticks. There was only one
other house around, and there was nothing to do but

count the cars that drove on by. It was a little closer to the mill, however, than the brick house, so I didn't have so far to ride in order to see my friends.

Dad continued drinking, finding his way to Gordon Road after work. Often he did not come home until the early morning hours. On one such occasion, it was about 2 o'clock in the morning, I awakened to some commotion outside my window. As I looked out, I saw the police in the yard behind my father, who had just gotten out of his car.

The officer asked my father for his license, and then, after he looked at it, gave it back. As he handed it over he said, "Okay, get in the car."

My father was slightly inebriated, but not incoherent. It wasn't uncommon for people to have a drink or two at a liquor house, do some socializing and then head home. He balked at the command. "What for?"

"Get in the car," the officer said again, ignoring my father's question.

"What for? What are you arresting me for?"

The policeman looked at him for a moment, but said nothing.

"Man, I'm home," my father continued, gesturing toward the house. "I don't know what you're arresting me for. Tell me what you're arresting me for."

The officer still said nothing, and my father turned and walked into the house, leaving him standing in our yard.

With all their talking back and forth, the whole house had awakened. As I watched my father enter the house, I could hear my mother moving about in the kitchen, preparing something for him to eat.

By this time, everyone was up and in the kitchen. We saw the policeman get into his car, and back up until he faced the house. All of a sudden, a blazing light flashed across my eyes. He'd turned his spotlight onto the house. Then there was a short screeching sound as the officer turned on a bullhorn. "McBride!" he bellowed. "McBride, come out!"

My father sat at the kitchen table eating a leg of fried chicken. He was quiet, but angry.

The officer repeated this command on for several minutes until my father abruptly stood up.

"Chick," my mother pleaded. "Just leave it be. Let him stay out there." She knew what was going on. She knew what would happen if he went outside. Then she turned to us. "Go on back to bed now, everybody." But there was no way we could just quietly go to sleep with all the commotion and tension.

But he would have none of that. Shaking her off, he emerged from the house with a piece of fried chicken in one hand and a knife hidden in the other. He headed straight for the officer, and I knew he was angry. He was just looking to get close to that policeman. The rest of us followed him out onto the porch, fearful of what would happen next.

As my father neared the policeman, I saw the officer was holding a shotgun, which he'd turned down toward the ground.

"What do you want with me?" my father yelled, still advancing on the policeman. "What did I do?" He took a bite of the chicken and waved it around, but kept the knife close to his trousers.

Just as my father came within a few feet of the policeman, two more police cars screeched up behind the first. Just then, the shotgun went off and everyone jumped. Briefly stunned by the loud noise, my father stopped in his tracks. Then the officers jumped my father, and as they wrestled him to the ground, they found the knife. I knew that if my father had reached that police officer, he would have used it.

"Watch it, Roy!" one yelled. "He's armed." They made a big scene out of the arrest.

As the policemen struggled with my father, Garfield stood beside me, fuming. He wanted to rush outside and jump into the fray, but our mother held him back as she tried to comfort the rest of us. I could see in her the concern for my father as he struggled with the policemen. Thoughts raced through my head, but I knew not to go outside. I stood and seethed as they put my father into the police car and whispered, "One day this is going to change."

News of my father's arrest reached the mill later that morning by the start of the workday. By the time he was released from jail, everyone knew he had been arrested for resisting arrest. Of course, we never knew why he was being arrested in the first place, but it didn't matter. The police had their excuse, and that's all they needed. In those days, you didn't ask the police to account for their actions, not if you were black, and so we never did.

My father's foreman had already decided to move him to work in another section, presumably as some sort of punishment for the arrest. When my father arrived at work, he was pegged as a troublemaker and told by his foreman he was being transferred. No questions, no discussions. It was a done deal, and my father had no say in it. But instead of complying, he quit in protest. He collected his retirement money and went home. That was the end of him working at the mill.

If times were difficult before my father was arrested, they were doubly so afterward. As a result, I often wondered how we were going to make it. My father was in his early 50s with no formal education, and so the jobs he could get were menial and did not pay enough to adequately support the family. But, he was a man who knew how to stand up for himself and his family, and he taught us by example. There was no color the night my father was arrested, no authority he was bowing to. He never feared anyone just because they were white. Someone had come onto his property and then tried to make him surrender himself without giving him even one justification for it. He knew that wasn't right. The only reason they were able to arrest him at all was because he was outnumbered.

Soon enough, the pension money ran out and we were forced to tighten our belts even more. Given our circumstances, it was understood that we would leave school by age 16 or 17 to go work in the mill. We had to move once again because the landlord wanted the house for one of his relatives. We moved around the corner from the mill, down on Gordon Road. Dad was doing odd jobs in the area trying to make ends meet. These were difficult times for the family and on many days, we did not know where our next meal was coming from.

Once on Gordon Road, my dad decided to open a liquor house. Since it was a home business, we were all involved in the production of the whiskey. Mom had to be home to sell the alcohol. Dad bought the white lightnin'—we called it scrap iron—from a "distributor." To create the golden whiskey color, he'd add some coloring to it and it looked just about like it was store bought. Then, along with our help, he bottled the finished product. Garfield, Eddie, Richard and I went around collecting empty bottles and caps, brought them home, and then cleaned and sterilized each one before filling them with the whiskey bought by our dad.

My father also made a type of beer called home brew. Our job was to find beer bottles for it. We filled the bottles and then capped them with a capper he bought, and put the finished product in the refrigerator. It was a clean little assembly line, and we did all right.

We would have done better except that Dad tended to consume his own supply, and often brought friends by to drink, too. Because he did not keep track of his inventory, he never knew how much supply he had, how much he sold, and how much he lost. Still, his efforts were in the right direction; he was trying to make something happen.

One of his ways of making things happen was to demand that I quit school and work with him. "Come on, go with me. I need your help," he said to me one day after he had been drinking. This was his way of telling me it was time for me to do as my brothers had done before me. At the time, he was working in the local pulp mill, which was hard, and at times dangerous work.

"I can't do that," I responded evenly.

"Why not?" He was surprised by my answer.

"I graduate from high school in a few months."

Now my father was stunned. He had no idea how

far along in my education I was. Although I was the fifth of eight children, I would be the first to graduate from high school. But my father had his mind fixed on making a living, not on education. "So you can't help me?" he demanded.

"No, I'm almost to graduation," I repeated, standing firm in the face of his anger.

When I refused to quit school, my father responded cruelly, "Then what good are you to me?"

I was too stunned to speak. "He would not say that to me," I thought. "The liquor is talking." I had my ideas about success, and about what my future would be. Neither of these included quitting school and hustling the way my father did to make ends meet. Furthermore, I saw myself as an example for my younger brothers since I was going to be the first one to graduate from high school. My father, however, was dealing with the pressures of making a living. His question hung in the air between us until we made a truce of sorts.

The confrontation about my quitting school cooled down after my father sobered up. Nothing more was said about my going to work with him. In the end, it was my father who, without being asked, bought me a brand-new suit for graduation. It was blue, and I knew I looked smart when I put it on for the first time.

Things were happening fast. With only a few weeks left before graduation, I ran into Miss Harriet Jones. She was a soft-spoken freshman, and someone I felt comfortable talking to in part because she was younger. The girls my age were intimidating, and I already knew Harriet a little.

Even though she was a quiet girl, she was nobody's fool. About a year previously I walked her home from school. I found out later that the house was not hers after all, and I figured that was her crafty but polite way of saying that she did not want to have anything to do with me. Since then, we had not spoken until the day we ran into each other. Literally. I was coming out of the lunchroom, which doubled as the auditorium, after practicing for graduation, when we bumped into each other.

"Oh!" we both exclaimed simultaneously as her purse fell to the ground. I knelt to pick it up for her, and, still on bended knee asked, "Are you all right?"

She gave me a small smile and took her purse. Her movements were efficient but fluid, friendly. Her smile was gracious, lingering just long enough for me to register her approval, but not any longer than that. "Thank you."

"Sorry about running into you," I said, but then reconsidered. She was very pretty, and I already knew from her ruse about her house that she was smart. "I mean, I'm not sorry that I am talking to you now, just sorry if I gave you a scare."

"No, I'm all right."

I pulled a piece of paper from the notebook I carried. "Here is my number. If you would like to go out sometime, give me a call," I said, scribbling down my information.

"Thank you, Cornell." Her smile was bigger this time.

She knows my name, I thought, grinning to myself.

We started going out shortly thereafter.

In the meantime, I wrote to some relatives to see if they could put me up. I'd grown up hearing about New York, the mythical land of streets paved with gold. It was the place where you were bound to find success— whatever that meant. The way I heard it, all you had to do was get there and you could not lose. There were jobs in New York that a black person just couldn't land in Georgia, or anywhere in the South. I could play base-ball, too, and land myself on a professional team. Friends, relatives and folks from the neighborhood who had been there always came back smiling, dressing smartly, and affecting with a strange accent. They even pretended that they couldn't stand the Southern heat and the bugs that wouldn't let you alone!

I graduated high school on June 6, 1961, with my proud parents in the audience. It was a big deal that they came to see me get my diploma. They were not expressive people, but having them there with big smiles on their faces was enough for me to know they felt I'd done right.

Somehow, I matured into a responsible teenager who wanted to complete his education and pave the way for his younger brothers to do the same. By the time I was 17, I had learned that I did not want my life to be limited to the mill. I did not know exactly what it was I *did* want, but it had to be something more, some-thing different. I knew that I could not end up the way others before me had, others I would see every day outside of school.

In my neighborhood where the bus dropped us off every day there was a tree where guys who'd already graduated or quit school would hang out all day long. Every day I got off the bus from school, and every day there they were, doing nothing but sitting under a tree. As I approached graduation, I knew I did not want to end up like them. I did not want to find myself under that tree. I vowed to myself that I would be out of Savannah before the new school year started in September.

There were other good reasons to leave the South. Tension and violence were increasing in a very public way. Ever since the international coverage of the brutal murder of 14-year-old Emmett Till in Mississippi in 1955 , the push for civil rights, and the groundswell of frustration over generations of oppression were reaching new heights all over the South. Though black people were not disappearing the way they were in Mississippi, and Georgia was not as rough as Mississippi, it was still the South, and I was a young black man with a propensity to speak my mind.

Young blacks were openly expressing themselves after being oppressed for so long. There was an awakening, and it took the form of verbal, and sometimes physical, expression. There was the desire to do more and have more than you thought you could ever have. The world was opening up. Life was more than the mill. There was rage that developed as things opened up. Having been raised to stand up for my beliefs, I could have become embroiled in the violence that came out of the various attempts at nonviolent confrontations. Some had already started thinking more militantly than what was happening in the movement, and when I saw the brutality all around me, I thought maybe we should get guns.

I had always been something of an individualist, and so had not joined the organized movements for civil rights, such as the SCLC or NAACP. But I was aware and I was interested. In high school I had a job at Food Town, a local market in Savannah, and would often take off my apron and head down the street to see what was happening. Sit-ins at Kresky's and Woolworth's drew large crowds, and I was often amongst them. We would mill about, waiting for something to happen, and sometimes incite an event by taunting and insulting the white crowds that gathered opposite us. Sometimes, when the fire hoses opened up on the blacks, I would get out just in time. The scenes were chaotic: police and firemen all over, whites and blacks forced at times to move shoulder to shoulder.

In the end, I left just in time. Had I stayed in the South, I most definitely would have become militant. As it was, my brothers and cousins became increasingly involved in the Civil Rights movement, and they landed in jail. The summer after I left Savannah, they were stuck in prison with the heat turned on full blast and no water to drink except what they could get after they cleaned out the commode. Police and citizens alike were criminals, and the line was often blurred between right and wrong.

Chapter 4: New York, New York!

Though it meant leaving behind my family and my new girlfriend, I decided to head up to New York. On August 20, 1961, I left Georgia for the first time and headed toward a new life.

I traveled with two friends—Lawrence Tate and Sam Smalls. Lawrence had a sister, Katie, in the Bronx, and he was going to stay with her. Sam and I were hoping to stay with my grandparents over on Lexington Avenue on the Lower East Side.

When we arrived in New York City, I was down to my last $2, and looking forward to a home-cooked meal at my grandparents' house. It had been raining steadily, and was dark by the time the bus pulled into the station. Katie was there to pick us up. As she dropped Sam and me off at my grandparents' place, she said, "If you run into a problem, call a taxi and come to 1054 Boston Road." Boston Road, in the Bronx, was where Katie lived with her husband, Ralph, and two daughters, Cynthia and Lolene. Katie was a wise woman who knew things probably weren't going to be like we thought, and she was right.

From the looks on my grandparents' faces when they opened their door, I don't think they were expecting me.

"Yes?" my grandmother said, not recognizing me as I stood there with Sam.

"Grandma, it's me! Cornell."

"Cornell? Our Cornell?" Before I could answer, she ushered us in and had us sit down. My grandfather was equally surprised to see us.

I'd seen my mother's parents only once in my life before that night, when I was about 10 years old. The Jones family had left the South in the mid-1940s, so my mother was the only member of the family who stayed behind. She was the oldest of the Jones children, and had married my father before her parents and younger siblings moved to New York. My mother and her family had remained in contact through letters written back and forth over the years, but since it was hard to arrange trips to visit, the letters were the only contact they'd had.

I could see they had a houseful of grandkids, cousins of mine I'd never met, along with one or two of my aunts and uncles. I knew then that there just wasn't going to be enough room for us.

"Why don't you try your Uncle Freeman and Aunt Ruby down the block?" my grandfather offered.

We did, but they had a very small apartment, and therefore could offer a place only for me.

As the night wore on, I realized that the impression I had about everyone in New York doing well, including my relatives, was far from the way things really were. I had thought it would be a simple matter of my writing to tell my grandparents that I was coming to New York, and that I would be received with open arms.

We called Katie around 11 o'clock that night. "Take a cab over," she said. I remember putting on my high school football letter-jacket just before we made a run for the cab. Even though it was August, there was a chill from all the rain that wouldn't seem to let up. When we arrived at her place, she came out and paid the fare. She knew we were down to our last dollars. Up to that point, my New York experience was not going well. But with Katie's generosity and guidance, things would soon turn around.

Katie and Ralph put us up at their place that night, and Lawrence, Sam and I stayed with her until I left New York almost two years later. She helped us get settled and eventually find jobs, and was a great support to me my first time so far from home. Katie counseled us about what we should and shouldn't do in New York. She and Ralph knew the city well, having lived there for many years, so she could tell us about negotiating the city, and being careful riding the subway and walking the streets.

Living at Katie's was home away from home. She did for me what I could not have imagined when I decided to move to New York City. She and Ralph were like parents to me—I was, after all, only 18 and on my own for the very first time, so having Katie and Ralph and their kids was like having a ready-made family. We pretty much had the run of the house, and though we pitched in to help with expenses, what we received far exceeded our contribution. We paid $8 a week for rent, but Katie fed us and even washed our clothes. She really looked after us, and I have always felt indebted to her for the help she gave me when I was a young man.

I looked for work right away, but it wasn't easy. New York was not paved with gold. Eventually, I bought a job. In those days, it was common to pay private employment services for job leads. For $20 they would send you out on jobs. I saw a sign in a window of an employment office on Third Street that read, "Jobs for Sale," so I went in and paid my $20.

The job I bought was at a pharmaceutical company in the Bronx called Davis and Edwards Pharmaceuticals. Though I moved up in the company, I quickly realized that working there would not get me the success I was seeking.

I had things to do and not a lot of time to get them done. With no money to my name when I started out in New York, my burning drive to make something of myself made me feel like I was wasting time every moment I wasn't striving toward my big break.

While I was in New York, Harriet and I kept in close contact, writing each other often. All the while I knew I was working to make our future better than it would be if I just went back to Savannah.

So, I turned my attention to baseball to see if I could make something out of that. There were various teams that played in the parks, and I went around to see if they needed players. I ended up with a ragtag bunch of guys. The team wasn't very good, and we didn't practice much, but we did play around a lot. One time I was pitching right next to Yankee Stadium. People watching the game were amazed by my curve ball. It was my only good pitch, so I pretty much had to use it. But I also knew that the higher up you got in the game, the better the players were, and these guys knew not to swing at my curve ball. My other pitches, however, weren't exceptional. One batter, a big, young white guy, kept fouling balls off me. Frustrated, I finally decided to throw one right past him. I reared back and threw the ball as hard as I could, and the guy knocked it out of the park. As I watched the ball sail over the fence, I thought, "Well, this isn't it. I want to be successful, but maybe it's not baseball." I knew it was time to leave New York.

"I'm going to join the Air Force," I told Katie one evening. "Nothing is happening for me here."

"I don't know, Cornell," she shook her head. "Now is not a good time. Don't you read the papers?"

"Of course I read the papers!"

She raised her eyebrows at me. "Well then, I guess

you know about the Cuban missile crisis?" Then her tone softened. "There are a lot of things goin' on, Cornell. I just don't want to see you get yourself into something you can't get out of."

"What else can I do? I am almost 20 years old, and what have I done? I need an education. I need skills."

"I did not tell Katie at the time, and maybe I did not realize it myself very clearly, but I was planning to make my life with Harriet, and I wanted to be ready to take on the responsibility of heading a household."

"After serving," I told Katie, "I can go to college. I have been here almost two years. It's time I move on." I also had other motivation, to fulfill the promise I had made to my mother to build her a house. That was not going to happen if I remained in New York working at dead-end jobs or chasing the illusion that I would play ball in the majors.

So I enlisted with the Air Force in November of 1962, the day President Kennedy announced the Cuban blockade, and went off to basic training in Texas. My first airplane ride ever was that trip to Lackland Air Force Base in San Antonio. It was excit-ing until one of the engines caught fire and we had to put down to change planes. Eventually, I made it to Lackland and through basic training. By that time, I felt I had some experience in the world. I felt more mature than most of the other guys, who were younger and away from home for the first time.

After completing basic training, I learned I would be stationed at the Air Force base in Plattsburgh, New

York. But before reporting for duty in January of 1963, I was given a short leave for the Christmas holiday and went to see my family and Harriet. I'd missed Harriet so much, and seeing her again made me appreciate her patience and support that much more.

"Let's get married next year," I said, "Then I'll be 21." I knew as I said it, though, that it would be hard to wait.

Chapter 5: Lonely in Plattsburgh

After spending the Christmas holidays at home with Harriet and the rest of my family, it was time for me to head to my permanent duty station in Plattsburgh, New York. Along the way I also paid a visit to Katie, Ralph and the rest of the gang.

When I left New York City, it was a clear winter day. The temperature was in the mid-40s, and there was not much snow on the ground. For some reason, I thought to myself that maybe the weather was going to get warmer as I traveled north. I guess I had not paid much attention to geography in high school because the farther north I traveled, the deeper the snow got and the lower the temperature dropped. By the time I arrived in Plattsburgh, it was snowing, dreary, and the temperature was hovering around freezing. Never in my life had I been so cold! I was chilled to my bones before I'd walked ten feet from the bus. New York City had been tropical compared to Plattsburgh. "What have I done?" I asked myself as the Plattsburgh air slapped me in the face.

The base's personnel office was warm and inviting, and I was more than happy to sign in.

"Go back outside, Airman," the personnel officer said.

"I beg your pardon?" I had only just started to feel my toes again, and this guy wanted to send me back out there in the freezing cold!

"Go outside, turn right, and you'll see a bus station. Catch the bus to your barrack."

I stared at him blankly.

A flicker of annoyance crossed his face. "Come here, I'll show you." I walked over to his side of the desk, where a window faced the area where I was to catch my bus.

"I don't see a thing," I said. There was nothing but snow. No bus stop was in sight, not even the one where I'd been let off to sign in.

"There," he pointed out into the white blur, but I could not see a thing, and I doubted he could, either. "Well," he said, frustrated by my inability to see the sign. "It's out there. Just go outside. The bus will show up."

So I turned up the collar of my Air Force blues, slung my duffel bag over my shoulder, and kept my head down against the wind. The storm was not looking like it would let up anytime soon, and I braced myself against the cold. A bus did arrive, and took me to my barrack on the other side of the base. First thing in the morning, I thought to myself as I headed toward the building against the barrage of snow, I'm going to find a way to get out of here.

Well, the next morning, I learned that I could get out

of my service, but it would be a Dishonorable Discharge. I would have none of that, and right away dropped the idea of leaving. Besides, leaving the Air Force would take me farther away from the promise I had made to my mother. So, I hunkered down against the cold and turned my attention to the job I'd come to do.

When I was asked at the end of basic training how I wanted to fulfill my service, I was given a number of options. What I never considered was how my options could affect my chances of being called up to fight in Vietnam, or would be affected by the Cuban missile crisis.   There was already talk of retraining Airmen for the Army, so I knew that if I got called up, there would not be much I could do about it. Instead, I thought about what I enjoyed, what I could learn more about and would excel at.

"I want to be a coach," I had said.

"Recreational Services," was the response. "Next!"

My specific assignment was in the Physical Conditioning Unit, and as a fitness instructor, my duty was to make sure that the personnel on the base was physically fit.

"All the pilots and other base personnel have to pass a physical fitness test call the 5 Basic Exercise Program (5BXbx)," I was told. "In addition, the pilots have to pass a self-defense test. It's your job to make sure every pilot is fit to fly and ready to engage in combat should they be shot down behind enemy lines and have to defend themselves." The defense course they took was called Combative Measures. Most of them, however, did not take the program seriously and could not fight their way out of a brown paper bag if they had to. In short order, it was clear to me that they did not plan to, either.

A captain said to me, "All this Combative Measures stuff is no use because if he was shot down, he would be dead anyway."

"So why are we doing this?"

"Because we have to."

"Why do we have to?"

"Air Force regulations."

"But nobody follows the regulations."

"That's not the point."

"Okay, then, what's the point?"

"Do what you have to do to make the system work. It's like this: The rules state that if a pilot fails his Combative Measures exam, he gets taken off flying status. If he gets taken off flying status, he's got to go back and be trained properly."

"Okay, so what's the problem with that?"

"The instructor," the captain continued pointing at me, "that means you, is held responsible for the pilot's failure because you are held responsible for his fitness in the first place."

"But I can't be responsible for his fitness," I protested. "Especially if he doesn't care about passing in the first place. That's crazy. That's like trying to make the horse drink."

"But that's the system. So, here's how you make it work. Since no instructors want to be held responsible for a failing pilot, make sure that no one's flying status is ever affected for lack of fitness."

"So you just push 'em on through," I said, with some disgust.

"Exactly. Then the Air Force thinks that there is a 100 % passing rate, even though that's impossible."

It was clear to me early on that the military was more concerned with form than with substance.

This system went against my ideals of hard work and accountability, but I knew better than to try to fight it. The United States Armed Services was not an organization I wanted to battle. Besides, promotion in the ranks depended on getting along, and bucking the system would not get me promoted. I had learned my lessons well growing up in Savannah where you had to learn to be accepting of things when you have no power to change them. I knew that I could only fight the battles I had a good chance of winning. Of course, being in possession of the good judgment to recognize when I had a good chance of winning had not been developed overnight.

So, instead of working against a system that was in no hurry of changing, I remembered my mother's words, and focused on how I could succeed in the future by spotting and creating opportunities for success. But I did continue to be lonely, and there *was* something I could do about that sooner than later.

When I first got to Plattsburgh, it was a difficult adjustment because there were few black residents in town, and not many on base, either. Consequently, there wasn't much nightlife, and so we often went up to Montreal—we called that "going up the trail." There was one black club in Plattsburgh called The House by the Side of the Road, and we sometimes would hang out there. But as a young airman, and a lowly one at that, the new environment was a little disorienting.

All that winter I thought of Harriet. As I trudged through the snow that winter in Plattsburgh, I knew I could not wait a year for us to get married. Almost 21 was good enough for me, and Harriet was already 18. I had to figure out a way to speed up the date of our marriage. It had been hard on both of us being apart, and even though money would be tight, at least we would be together. So Harriet came up to New York in July of 1963, and Harriet and I were married.

At that time, families of enlisted men were not provided housing on the base, and most definitely not the family of an airman 2nd class. You had to be a sergeant or have four or more years of service to land base housing for a family. So Harriet and I moved into a small apartment in Plattsburgh. It was not particularly nice, and for all that not even easy to land. There were people who did not want to rent an apartment to me, but from their behavior, it was only a hunch on my part that it was because of the color of my skin. But I was so happy to have Harriet with me that I did not dwell on it for too long. Besides, soon enough, the reality of family life set in, and that distracted me from the subtle racism of those few people I had encountered while searching for an apartment.

I was a married man, and family was upon us: Sheila McBride, our beautiful baby girl, was born.

Soon enough, I made some time, and I began writing to the State Human Rights Commission to complain about the difficulties we were having with securing decent housing. Through these letters, the local paper, the *Plattsburgh Press Republican*, noticed our plight. They ran a story on our housing odyssey.

Fortunately, someone who read the article came forward and offered us a four-room bungalow on Route 9. Though in disrepair when we found it, this place at least had the promise of livability. After Harriet and I worked on it inside and out, we finally had a decent place to live.

It soon became clear that not only was housing a problem, but so was money. Even after I took on another job, we were having trouble making ends meet. Harriet started working a little, and we started to get on our feet, financially. Soon enough, we had more good news: Harriet was pregnant again. Though this would force us to rethink her working and our living situation, it was wonderful news. After discussing our options, we agreed that we could no longer afford the cottage. Harriet would return to Savannah with Sheila during her pregnancy, and I would move back on base and into the barracks.

Later that year, it was time to bring my family back together. On a brief leave in the spring, I drove down to Savannah to pick up my family and bring them back with me once again to Plattsburgh. Money was still tight, but we wanted to be together for the birth of our second child. Just how difficult things were for us financially did not hit home for me until I was at my parents' house.

"Cornell," my mother asked one day as she worked in the kitchen preparing supper. "I need a few things from the store. Would you go for me?"

As soon as she handed me the list, my heart raced and my face burned with shame. I did not have enough gas in my car, having just made it to Savannah with the last of my cash, and would not be receiving my next paycheck for several days. One of my buddies had agreed to send it down to me so I would have money for the return trip, but at the moment, I was stuck.

My parents had no indoor bathroom, and were scraping by, and there I was about to tell her I could not even get to the store for her. They thought I was doing well. After all, they had a son in the military who had a family of his own. How could I tell her I didn't have enough money to put gas in my car?

I was ashamed that I had not succeeded. I was ashamed that I was not able to take care of my mother. What had I been doing all this time? What had I accomplished?

I could barely open my mouth to speak, my mouth was so dry. "Mom," I said.

"Mm-hmm," she answered absent-mindedly, focused as she was on her work.

"I, uh, I'm waiting on a check in the mail. But right now, I'm clean out of gas to get to the store."

"Okay," she said, without missing a beat. She reached in her bosom and pulled out a handkerchief with the money tied into a knot, and as she untied the money my heart sank and I felt ashamed. My mother gave me the $2 needed for the gas, and I went off, humiliated, to the market.

I resolved never again to be in this position. When Harriet, Sheila and I returned to Plattsburgh, things were going to be different. I was going to make things happen. We were going to get ahead. We were going to succeed. I would sign up for classes on base, so I could prepare for college, and I would work as many jobs as there were hours to work. I had worked part-time at the Officer's Club on base, but that income was not nearly enough to accomplish the financial success I had in mind.

As we headed back to Plattsburgh, the weather was clear, and the air cool and dry—a perfect day for driving. So determined was I to change my life, I could not get us back to Plattsburgh fast enough. I was a man on a mission.

Soon after we crossed into South Carolina, Harriet needed to stop for the restroom, and so I decided to stop at a Shell station up ahead that looked to be open. I figured I would fill the tank. I didn't really need gas, but I did not want to go to a business and ask to use their bathroom without buying anything.

We pulled up in front of the pumps, and the white attendant, a doughy looking man of about 40, came out. "Can I help you?" he asked with a hint of suspicion in his voice.

"Yeah, will you top it off?"

He worked his jaw for a moment, as if deciding what to do, and then silently yanked the handle from its cradle.

"Say," I asked, "my wife needs the restroom. Do you have a key?"

Without looking up, he said, "Yeah, get the key from one of them boys over there," and gestured toward the garage where a couple of black guys were working on a car. As I walked over to them to ask for the key, Harriet secured Sheila in her seat, and then followed just a few paces behind.

"Guy says you all have a bathroom key," I called out. "For my wife," I explained. As I approached them, they looked up at me, and then saw Harriet. "Man," one of them said slowly, "she can't go in that old colored bathroom around back."

At once, I knew exactly what he meant. He was warning me that the "colored" bathroom was not fit for any human, let alone a pregnant woman. I was furious. I stormed past Harriet back to the attendant, who was pumping my gas. "I don't want the key to no colored bathroom! Give me the key to the regular bathroom. Right now!"

His pudgy face suddenly froze in shock. Then a look of pure hatred washed over him, freezing into a cold stare. "You wait a minute here!" he shouted at me, as if to put me in my place, and then turned to go inside the station.

Somehow I knew he was going to get his gun and would probably shoot me. I stood there with nothing, my wife behind me and my baby daughter in the car. So I quickly followed him into the store not knowing what to expect, and wondering how I was going to get out of this situation.

I stood at the cash register, waiting, and he reappeared from the back room. I was right, he did have a gun, and he was striding right at me. Knowing I had hardly any choices at all, I stood there, waiting for him to come to me. In my left hand, I held the money I had ready to pay for the gas. In order to diffuse the situation, and without a word, I handed him the money so he would take it with his right hand—and he did! He put the gun down and reached out for the money, while muttering insults under his breath. Then I turned and hustled out the screen door, which slapped against the frame behind me.

"Come on," I hissed at Harriet as I reached the car. "We've got to go!" With Harriet and I safely in the car, we took off out of there as fast as we could. Harriet never did get to use the bathroom there, but we soon found somewhere else to go. I was angry about the incident for a long time, and wrote to Shell to complain about the way my wife and I had been treated and then threatened with a gun, while our baby daughter was barely 50 feet away. They wrote back and said they had no control over their franchises, but that they regretted what had happened. I did not use a Shell station for years afterward.

As we left the station, I was on fire, a mix of anger, shame and determination. Never again would I stand for having no money or being treated like a subhuman. I headed north, determined to change my life, and New York was the place where I would do it.

New York was more progressive than the South. In the South, prejudiced white people were more open about their belief in their own superiority. In New York there was a history of progressive social movements and attitudes, and more industry and career opportunities than in the South. From the old abolitionist movements to the diversity that grew out of the immigrant population, New York seemed to me a place where a young black man could make something of himself.

I was hopeful, but I wasn't naïve. I had already experienced racism when seeking housing for my family and me. I wasn't the same 18-year-old who went to New York City for the first time thinking the streets were paved with gold and folks treated each other equally and with respect. Instead, I was a cautiously optimistic young man with a pregnant wife and child, looking forward to getting back to my service and the path to future success. So as we drove on to New York after leaving South Carolina, my motivation was renewed, and my anger at myself subsided. But had I known about the racism I was about to experience, I may have driven just a little bit slower.

Chapter 6: Plattsburgh "Progressiveness"

Back in New York with Harriet and Sheila, we found a cottage where we could live temporarily while I set about finding suitable housing for us. Every day I circled "For Rent" ads in the paper. I called on places to set up viewing appointments, or went directly to an address if it was listed in the ad. Most often, my family and I would be dismissed politely. People would smile and say apologetically, "Oh, I'm so sorry, it's just been rented." Then they quickly removed the rental sign that was sitting in front of the building. It turned out there were a lot of places that I lost out on because someone else supposedly had gotten there first.

They sounded so genuine that, in the beginning, I thought they were on the level. They did not seem to be discriminating against me the way that others had. But then, as I continued to search the papers for suitable apartments, I began to notice that many of the listings were places I'd gone to see—the very places I was told had already been rented. So I called on them again, but this time I wore the nice blue suit my father

had given me for my high school graduation. Maybe I
didn't look presentable enough, I thought. If I look like
a businessman, if I look like a success, they'll rent to
me. They didn't. As I later told a reporter from the
Plattsburgh Press Republican, "In the South they don't
hide their prejudice. Here, if your black skin offends
them, you get the stall and the runaround." It would-
n't have mattered to them if I'd driven up in a Rolls
Royce. They were not going to rent to me simply
because I was black. I realized it was not just a few
people who had this attitude; it was rampant.

Sometimes, people accidentally revealed their true
feelings, as happened one time when I called on an
apartment on South Catherine Street, and then when I
arrived to see it, no one was there. I waited an hour,
but the woman who I was supposed to meet never
showed up. Later, I called to find out what happened.
The woman stammered, and then blurted out, "But
you're a *Negro!*" From speaking to me on the phone,
she had expected to see a white man.

Other times, people were more direct in their prejudice, but it was not as common as the lies I was told.
I did have several doors slammed in my face. One man
told me he did not want any Negroes in his neighborhood. He was sorry, but if one of "us" moved in, soon
the whole neighborhood would go Negro.

Some of my white friends in Plattsburgh were told
by landlords that renting to blacks would drive the
whites out of the community. It was like they thought
we had some sort of infection they might catch if they
got too close to us. My white friends were also told
that black people are "hard" on property, and so the

upkeep for landlords was too expensive. But the available housing was already in terrible disrepair. The house we used to live in on Route 9 we had improved tremendously, but that did not seem to matter. The thinking seemed to be, if you lived in a run-down place, it was your fault.

My search for decent housing lasted a year, and during that time I sent at least a half-dozen complaints to the State Commission on Human Rights. There was no legitimate reason for landlords not to rent to my family and me. Our housing situation, however, did not improve. We were forced to live in less than acceptable accommodations simply because no white owners of nice places would rent to us—and it was not as if we were trying to rent beyond our means. We always looked at rentals that were advertised within our price range, and we were scrupulous about our budget. With my income as our only source of revenue, we weren't about to try living somewhere we could not afford. Later, after Harriet gave birth to our second child, she would work on base in the nursery, but at the time she already had enough work at home.

Word of my campaign to unmask racial prejudice in the housing market began to get out. Depending on whom you asked, I was gaining either notoriety or popularity. It seemed that people were divided over my actions, some standing squarely behind me, and others taking the opposite side. Soon enough, I was feeling like a marked man. There were some white airmen and officers on base who did not approve of my activism. They didn't care that I was simply trying to protect my family. I was labeled a troublemaker and there were efforts to discredit me, apparently as a means of ultimately silencing me.

Other whites simply thought I was making a big deal out of nothing. But this was not a battle I could walk away from, regardless of whether standing up to discrimination branded me as a troublemaker. I did not ask for the attention, and I surely did not ask for a fight. But I was backed into a corner, and there is no motivation quite like protecting your family to take on all comers. I was already motivated to succeed, and now I was motivated to protect my family and remove the obstacles to my success. If I could not go around them, I was determined to go over or through them. Once it was started, I was not going to back down, whether or not that got me on the bad side of some of my supervisors.

Many of my fellow black airmen were not behind me. Though there was not a large black population in Plattsburgh, and even less on the base (about 20 % of the servicemen in the Air Force was black), most were disinterested in changing the housing situation. I chalked their attitude up to resignation. They just wanted to keep their heads down and make it through unscathed, and in some ways I couldn't blame them. The military institution itself was not an organization of swift changes. There was one officer, a black master sergeant, I distinctly recall because he did not want anyone to know he was a supporter of the civil rights movement. I, on the other hand, always spoke my mind. My mother and father always told me, "If you don't stand for something, you will fall for anything."

Among those who scorned me or gave me flak was my immediate supervisor in charge, Sergeant Landau, a wormy-looking white guy who always seemed to be compensating for something he thought he lacked. He gave me my very first (and last) poor performance report. Apparently, Sergeant Landau filed the report rather abruptly—seemingly out of nowhere—and against regulations. All such reports were supposed to be viewed and witnessed by the person being reviewed. I never saw my evaluation until I learned about it through one of my friends who worked in Personnel.

"Say, Mac," he said. "Why do you have a bad report?"

"What? What are you talking about?"

"I just filed it the other day. And," he said, raising his eyebrows, "your signature is not on it."

"That's not right," I said, and turned to find out what had happened. "Thanks, man. Thanks a lot."

I pursued a meeting with the higher-ups, which led to a confrontation in front of my squadron commander, a burly, no-nonsense career military man.

"Sergeant Landau," my squadron commander asked, "How do you explain this low rating for Airman McBride?"

"Poor performance," he shrugged noncommittally.

"What sort of poor performance?" The squadron commander leafed through my file. "Look here, there are consistent 9s and 10s on performance reports, and then suddenly, and without explanation, the numbers suddenly dropped. Was there any kind of reprimand beforehand?"

"No," Landau replied. He had no plausible explanation for my sudden and precipitous drop. Nor could he explain why I was not even informed of the report in the first place.

The report was discredited and removed, but it was clear to me that I was fighting two battles: one for my family, and one for myself. I was not about to allow anyone with power over my career ruin my chances of getting promoted. There was no way I could get promoted with 4s and 5s on my performance reports. Anyone who wanted to be promoted needed 9s and 10s—preferably the latter. Had I not stood up for myself, I could have been driven right out of the Air Force by superiors who could trump up charges against me, or make my life so miserable that there would be no point in staying. One airman advised me to "watch how fast you drive on base." My enemies would put up any smokescreen they could as a pretense to undermine me.

Fortunately, I did have good friends who were white and others who were black. That was one of the good aspects of the military. It brought black and white together. Previously, I had no friendships to speak of with white people. My whole life, even during my time in New York City, I had remained largely in the company of black people. I definitely never roomed with any of them, but I did in the Air Force. In the South, where segregation reigned, I grew up in an atmosphere that fostered mistrust of white people. In the Air Force, however, I made several very good friends who were white. So good, in fact, that they stood up for me when they could have just walked away.

Before I got married, some of the guys and I would

go out sometimes to The House By The Side of The
Road, (a black club) or another club, Brody's (a white
club). Once, at Brody's, my friends Carl and Dorazio
stepped in to help me after some white guys got mad
at me for talking to a couple of white girls. I was the
only black guy in the club, and probably would have
been hammered if Carl and Dorazio hadn't been there.
So, by the time I was embroiled in proving my housing discrimination experience, I had a number of
friends I could count on to support me.

One of those very good friends was Rudy Holmes.
He was a career military man who would make the
rank of senior master sergeant before he retired, but he
wasn't cut from the same cloth as many of the others
I'd come to know. When I met him, he'd just arrived
from a station overseas, and he brought with him a
European attitude and flair. Clean cut, athletic and
about six or seven years older than I, we became
friends while working in the same duty section.

Rudy thought of me as his little brother—he called
me "Corn"—and helped me enormously in my efforts
to prove discrimination. It was Rudy who helped me
write my letters to the Human Rights Commission, and
everything he did for me he did without concern for
himself. He risked his neck more than once, which is
saying a lot; it says more so if you were a career military man, and even more if you were someone like
Rudy, who wasn't the "keep your head down and nose
clean" sort of military guy. Rudy wasn't afraid. Instead,
he believed in knowing military regulations so that you
knew exactly what you could and could not do. This
was valuable knowledge, as I would soon learn.

Through the stories that ran in the local papers, and by word of mouth, my squadron commander learned of my travails. About the same time, Rudy and I found out that if a town discriminates against military personnel, the base commander can declare the town off limits to the base. What this would mean is that no one on base would be allowed to shop, or do business with the town. Of course, that would be the last thing he would want to do, and certainly no Plattsburgh officials would want that. He could also find housing for my family on base, but I already knew that was a stretch. Airmen 2nd Class just did not live on base. Nor did the base commander want the publicity that was increasingly kicking up all around me.

Soon enough, I was summoned to the base commander's office.

"Airman McBride," the base commander started. He was about 40, lean and wiry, with weathered skin. "We need to resolve this situation," he barked. "I don't like conflict on or surrounding my base."

"Yes, Sir," I agreed. "Nor do I. I just want my family to have the same opportunity as anybody else. I am not asking for anything I cannot afford."

"The only way I can help you is if we have proof you're being discriminated against. Do you have that proof?"

"No, Sir," I confessed. "Nothing but what I can tell you and what is in the papers."

"I think we can catch them in the act," my squadron commander said. "Then there will be proof."

"All right," the base commander said, dismissing us. "Take care of it."

I did not know precisely what that action would be, nor did I know how my efforts would turn out given how divisive my personal situation had become on base. It was then that I was reminded of my father. No matter what was happening around us when I was a child, my father always made me feel safe. He protected his family in difficult times, and I grew up in that security.

Now it was my turn to protect my family, to provide an environment in which my child, Sheila, and the infant we would soon welcome into the world would feel completely safe and cared for. The uncertainty of the future was no excuse not to take action, and I knew I was in the right. But I also knew that I could accept the consequences of my actions because my actions were right to begin with. It wasn't that I was in the wrong but trying to force it to be right. I had considered my options. When I was a willful child, I used to think I was always right. Then my father stopped me in my tracks. "When you think you're so right about something, stop and put yourself in the other person's shoes." I'd done that, and in the end, the shoes that mattered were those of my family. I would be right no matter what happened, and so I went ahead. When the *Plattsburgh Press Republican* reporter asked whether I preferred to the open prejudice of the South to the indirect prejudice I found in Plattsburgh, I responded, "That's a fine choice, isn't it?" It was not a choice I wanted my children to have to make.

The sting operation was simple: Along with one of my white sergeants, I would call on an apartment listed for rent. Then, if I were told the apartment had already been rented, my sergeant would come later to see if they would rent to him. If they did, my case would be proven. But if, instead, the property was later found to still be on the market, my claims would be found to be true. It did not take long for me to prove my case. The base commander finally decided the best option he had was to move my family and me onto the base. An Airman 2nd Class living on base! It was remarkable. That triumph was made all the happier when our family grew to four in August of 1965— Cornell Jr. was born.

Chapter 7: A Budding Entrepreneur

The publicity I received from the stories brought me to the attention of the only and very powerful black activist in Plattsburgh, and few white liberals living in Plattsburgh. The experience also brought me into contact with some remarkable people, including Jackie Archer, the president of the local NAACP. Hers was the one prominent black family in Plattsburgh, and she and her husband, Lloyd, readily accepted me and my family into theirs. We were invited to parties and other social events, and Jackie stepped in on several occasions to support me. Having Jackie on my side was one of the beneficial consequences of my taking action on the housing discrimination.

Jackie was a remarkable woman. A graduate of Spellman College in the early 1940s, Jackie was well ahead of her time. She moved her family to Plattsburgh to head up the local chapter of the NAACP shortly before I began my service at the Air Force base there. Jackie became a well-known figure for more than 30 years, working tirelessly to make life better for those whose lives were hard enough. If there was a problem for any minority—one did not have to be black to get help from Jackie—she was in there trying to make it right.

She helped me with my college work, too. I took an English 101 course at Plattsburgh University that focused on writing. This was an especially difficult course for me because I'd never done much writing, but I knew I would need this skill in the future. So, I dedicated myself to improving my writing. Every paper that I wrote came back with an "F" on it. Frustrated, but motivated to succeed, I went to the instructor for help. Instead, I got advice. "Son, college isn't for everybody, you know." I went directly to Jackie for help, and managed to pull my final grade up to a "D." It turned out to be the only "D" on my college record. I kept up with Jackie until she died, and still keep in touch with Lloyd. Though they divorced sometime after my family and I left Plattsburgh, I remained friends with them both.

Lloyd was the first black man who showed me, as an adult, how to be successful in business. Because I spent time socially with both Jackie and Lloyd, I came to know him fairly well, and we would talk at times about my future. I was still wandering then, trying to figure out how I was going to make my mark as a man, how I was going to create a comfortable life for my family, and how I was going to make enough money to build my mother the house I'd promised her. At a time when the average income for a family was $3,000 a year, I told Lloyd that I planned to make $10,000. Lloyd turned to me and said, "Mac, you're a better, smarter man. You can make a lot more."

I was so impressed that this successful businessman would take time to talk to me about life and business. After all, I was a young, lowly airman struggling to provide for my family. Why should he bother with me? To have a mentor such as Lloyd was invaluable, and he not only raised and broadened the standard of success I had in mind, but also showed me that I could—and should—influence others by my success. As Lloyd had done for me, I would someday do for others.

I'd been working hard to support my new family, but I knew that I needed to do more. The long period spent looking for housing and then fighting the discrimination I endured had, in some sense taken me away from my goal, but in another sense it reinforced the confidence I had to go out and succeed. I had picked a battle I believed I could win, and I won it. Now I needed to cultivate my mind with an education so that I could strengthen that confidence.

"We're laying the foundation for our next step," I said to Harriet. That next step was for me to go to college after completing my service. There was no question that a college education was going to open doors for a career in a way that would likely not be possible without it. I already had entrepreneurial instincts and interests, but I knew I had to develop study, organizational and intellectual skills, so that whatever career I chose, I would be qualified to succeed and prosper. So I studied for college, prepared for the SAT exam, did my service and started my own business. Harriet worked at the nursery center at the base, so she could take care of Sheila and Cornell Jr. at the same time.

"First thing," I said, "is we have to put ourselves on a strict budget—even stricter than before." Not only did we have to pay our bills, but we also had to put money away. With our goal clearly in mind, our immediate focus was to save money. "The G.I. bill will cover tuition costs for the academic year, but we'll still need money to live."

Harriet and I soon knew to the penny how much I would need to cover all our costs: rent, food, medical, gas and so forth. We did not eat out or go for drinks. As a young couple, we liked clubs and listening to music as much as anyone else, but if there was no money for it, we didn't go—and there was rarely, if ever, any money for it!

With two years of service left, I knew I had to act fast to get ahead. I got a job at Brody's, the local bar and restaurant frequented mostly by white officers. I also focused on a new business. It was a janitorial service I started on base with my good friend, Carl Wernett, and we hired three other friends to help. Carl was one of my best friends. We had gone through basic training together, had lived in the barracks together, and were about the same age and rank. If I didn't go up to Montreal or over to The House by the Side of the Road, I'd hang out with Carl over at Brody's. He introduced me to country music, and I introduced him to soul. I even came to like country music! Roy Orbison was one of my favorites. Carl was an unaffected guy from New Jersey, someone in whom I could not detect even the slightest hint of prejudice. He was simply devoid of any of that kind of hate.

Ours was the first business I'd started as an adult, and it brought me back to my days as a young entrepreneur in Georgia. I was creative and eager to learn how to run the most successful and excellent business in Plattsburgh.

Our business focused on cleaning the residences of people moving off the base. Most often, they did not have time to clean their housing, let alone stay around the base until the place passed inspection. Anyone living on the base had to leave his abode in excellent condition. But if you were being transferred, you didn't have time to clean up. That's where our service came in.

We advertised in the base circular, and soon had our first job. It took the five of us 100 hours to clean our first house! We weren't organized. We played around too much, and had no system for efficiently, but thoroughly, cleaning houses. After that first job, the others quit, and Carl and I were left with the business. We trimmed things down significantly on our next job, completing the cleaning in 20 hours. Soon enough, we were averaging two to three houses a week at $50 to $60 a house. That was a lot of money in those days, and more than we were making in the military. This was a second, or even third job for us, and so that number wasn't bad at all.

I took the business when Carl was transferred to Texas for three months, where they needed more physical training instructors. When he returned, he was no longer interested in our business, but I was.

"This is my opportunity to learn as much as I can about how to grow and maintain a quality business," I told Harriet one night over dinner. "I want to develop a reputation for excellence."

With each job, I learned how to become more efficient while maintaining the high quality for which I was becoming known throughout the base. For example, I learned how to prioritize the steps in the process so that I would simultaneously maximize efficiency. At each house, I would do a walk-through to determine the order of cleaning, and the order of cleaning was determined by the length of time required for each part of the house. Everything I did allowed me to do something else at the same time. I saturated the tile floors with stripper, and then went off to put the blinds in the tub to soak, while coating the oven with oven cleaner. Then I would work on the walls, cleaning off marks and scuffs, before moving on to the windows. With those done, I could turn my attention back to the floors, and so on.

My successes meant I could become more selective in choosing my clientele, and this was no small matter. If I was not sought after, I would have to take on jobs that would drain my time and efficiency, and so also my profit. A filthy house took twice as much time as one in relatively good condition. Given the choice, I took the nicer house so I could clean it and another, rather than spend all my time on the dirty one.

When I was asked to give a quote on a house, if it was particularly dirty, and therefore not a house I wanted to clean, I quickly calculated the amount of time it would take, and factored that into my quote.

The worse the condition of the house, the higher the price had to be for me to clean it. This approach to pricing helped me to eliminate clientele. As my business reputation grew, base housing inspectors put my name out around town. I recall one businessman calling me to look at a building he wanted cleaned, but I had to turn him down on the spot. Just from the walk-through, I could estimate the amount of time it would take to do the job, and so I gave him an estimate on the spot, figuring he would not take it. He didn't.

I must admit that this was a difficult lesson to learn, but I am glad I learned it early, when I was still a child. As a kid mowing lawns and doing odd jobs, I would often let the customer pay me what he thought the job was worth because I did not know. More often than not, I was underpaid. Part of my reticence was due to fear. Instead of focusing on what the job would take in time and manpower to complete, and then letting those criteria, along with a comparison of comparable businesses' rates determine my pricing, I simply feared asking for money. I feared the rejection that might come from someone balking at what I charged. So I sidestepped the issue, and in doing so, I lost out. Working hard is a fine and good thing, but one should not work for less than what he or she is worth, and certainly not for less than what the job is worth.

By the time I had the janitorial service to myself, I learned how to price houses. I had done market research so I could be competitive with other cleaning businesses, and then I did them one better by being so good. In this way, I could keep my rates up when I did agree to cleaning dirtier houses, and still make the same amount per hour as I would doing jobs that required less time. Once I had determined the profit I could reasonably expect to make, I set my rates so that I could keep my quality high and my quantity of jobs low. In the time I had my business, I learned a lot about how to function successfully in a service industry, and was keen to take that knowledge and build on it in another capacity.

Not everyone I knew had the same business drive and ethics as I. I recall asking my friend, Rudy Holmes, if he wanted to come clean houses with me.

"Clean houses?" he sniffed.

"I'm doing all right," I replied. "Besides, you're always borrowing money from me. Why not just earn your own?"

"If I have to make a living cleaning houses, then I choose not to make a living at all."

Rudy was a good friend. He'd been with me through my letter-writing campaign. His first son's birth was three days apart from Cornell Jr., and we were always very close. But we had very different ideas about work.

I told him, "At the end of the day, when a man goes to the store, all people care about is how he's going to pay. It doesn't matter if he's wearing a suit or overalls." I wore my overalls proudly, not just because I had built a business from the ground up while I was still in my early 20s, and not just because I did it while taking care of a family and serving my country in the Air Force, but because I did it *well*. The quality of my work, the excellence I strove everyday to achieve, was inextricable from the work itself.

One of my fondest memories of my business was going to the bank with my passbook each week to deposit money. It wasn't long before I became a known entity at the bank.

"Hello, Mr. McBride," tellers would greet me. They were happy to have my money, and I was happy to be saving it.

The discipline and focus established early on was paying off. It was no surprise to Harriet and me that sticking to our plan was starting to yield its rewards, and the more we saved, the more we wanted to save. These days, saving is an unusual (and for some, an almost impossible) idea. It seems that, no sooner do people have money, they spend it—and not on the necessities of life. Money is spent, to my mind, frivolously, and without regard for a future. Though we were very young, Harriet and I were money-wise and did not lose focus on our goal. Being financially successful is not about being smart. You can be mediocre, but if you're disciplined, you can find money you never thought was there.

By the time I completed my service to the Air Force, I'd saved $3,000 from the janitorial service and paid off all my debts, including the two cars Harriet and I had bought for the business and for her to get around. My company was so successful that the cleaning process I used was later adopted as standard military procedure for base housecleaning. I also learned about the importance of interpersonal relationships in business through my dealings with the base inspectors. I got to know all of them, and after a while, they knew they could trust me to make a house fit for inspection. My taking responsibility for the condition of the house allowed the tenant to clear the base before inspection, something not previously permitted. Because of its efficiency, this practice also became part of the military standard. Before then, people were not permitted to leave before inspection, and if the house did not pass, the tenant did not leave. This caused delays and problems down the line when a transfer was supposed to happen quickly.

As my discharge date in November of 1966 grew near, I began to look around New York for a college. I knew I needed my bachelor degree, and I wanted to have an education that would help me develop and hone my intellectual skills for a successful business career. But the schools that interested me were too expensive—beyond the range of what my G. I. Bill would cover. I knew I'd have to work anyway to support my family beyond the $3,000 I'd saved, and it would be almost impossible to work still more than that to cover books and tuition at an expensive school. At the same time, I did not want to return to Savannah, where I might easily be distracted by the proximity to home. We did know that we wanted to go back to the South, and so focused our attention on finding a suitable school there.

"We could stay here," Harriet offered. "We're doing alright."

It was true. We had a nice place to live, money, two cars and a color television. "I do not want to just do 'alright,'" I countered. "I want to *excel*. Whatever we grew up thinking was good enough can still be better. We just have to plan and be open to opportunity."

Harriet listened, and in the end agreed.

While figuring out what to do next, I learned that I could extend my service time for nine months with the intent to re-enlist. Extending my service would mean several things. First, instead of starting college in January, I could work for another nine months to earn more money, be discharged in July of 1967, and instead begin college the following fall. Second, service in excess of four years meant I could be upgraded to Airman 1st Class and receive an extra stripe. Third, servicemen with four-plus years of service were relocated to their state of origin, the state in which they first enlisted. This meant that movers packed up your belongings and drove them to your new home. Though my state of origin was New York, I did the calculations and saw that it would be much cheaper to simply pay the movers the cost of mileage, rather than either moving our things ourselves, or paying a moving company outright.

The nine-month extension did not commit me to re-enlisting, and though Harriet and I discussed the possibility of making a career in the military, I concluded that it would not give me the opportunities for advancement that I desired. I'd been in the military long enough to have learned that there are ways to make the system work for you—the nine-month extension being one way to take advantage of a great opportunity—but I wanted to make my own system. Nine months more service was beneficial, but I did not want anymore from the military after that.

Shortly after, I found out that an old high school teacher I admired, Mr. Malcolm Blount, was now at Fort Valley College in Fort Valley, Georgia.

"I found a school," I declared proudly to Harriet. "And it's in Georgia."

It looked to be a perfect fit, and much had changed in the time I had been away. I saw opportunities in the South that were never there before. So, in 1967, we headed back to Georgia. I was 24, married, a father of two, a businessman, activist and veteran. But there was still much to do.

Chapter 8: Hello, Afro!

Fort Valley was a small, typically Southern town. You could drive through its center in under two minutes. As we came to a stop at a light near its center, I turned to Harriet and said teasingly, "Well, this is home."

Without a word she looked around, and after taking in the meager surroundings, tears began streaming down her cheeks. We rolled on until we got to the house I had secured for us. When she got out and saw that it was right across the street from the town's funeral home, she got back in the car.

"What are you doing?" I asked, getting back into the car. "Let's get settled."

"I am not staying there," she declared adamantly, her eyes fixed on the funeral home. "Not one night."

So, we didn't. Instead, I bought a trailer with some of the $3,000 I had saved in Plattsburgh, which we decided would be the most economical living accommodations while I worked on my bachelor's degree. I convinced a local businessman Joseph Henry, who later became a friend of mine, to let me park it on his lot. Harriet and the kids and I quickly settled into our new life.

I also started growing out my hair.

After years of a military buzz cut, I was ready for a change. Besides, most of the young guys in the late '60s were sporting fine Afros, and I wanted one, too.

"Check this out," I said to Harriet one afternoon shortly before school started for the year. I patted the top of my head lightly and smiled. "It is growing, isn't it?" I said proudly.

Right away, Harriet understood. "Let me take a look."

I bent my head a little so she could inspect my budding Afro. From the corner of my eye I could see her dutifully measuring the length of my hair.

"Mm-hmm," she nodded. "In a little while, it'll be long enough for me to braid. That will help it stand up."

I smiled, and turned to the mirror to admire my hair. My hair will stand up, and I will stand out, I thought, smiling to myself.

I would stand out, indeed. I was on to a college career and a bright future for my family and me. I began classes in the fall of 1967 thinking I would study to become a poultry farmer. I would finally make up for the disappointments of my childhood attempt to raise turkeys and buy a hog to start a hog farm in my backyard!

Being a college student was exhilarating. I felt confident and capable. I knew I belonged there. I knew I was headed for a successful future. Having the maturity gained from service in the Air Force didn't hurt, either. I was several years older than my fellow college students, and appreciated the enormous changes the South had undergone in my six-year absence, from the

Voter's Rights Act, to the Civil Rights Act and to open housing. The atmosphere on campus was in step with the times: we felt free in a way they never before thought possible, and we took advantage of it. I was determined to learn as much as I could, and though I could not participate fully in college life, I did take on the outward appearance of my generation: I started wearing bell-bottoms and kept at growing out my Afro. It did not grow as big as I would have liked, and my hair could have been softer, but eventually the Afro became large enough to be noticeable.

I started out studying poultry management, but soon switched over to animal science, which served as a prerequisite to veterinary medicine. Colleges were recruiting qualified black students aggressively in those days, and so there were many opportunities available.

Among the other colleges recruiting in Georgia at the time was Mercer University up in Atlanta. My biology professor, Dr. Corker, organized a talk on Mercer's pharmacy studies program. Those of us who decided to take advantage of the opportunity to study at Mercer University's College of Pharmacy would be the vanguard of black pharmacists in the South. In 1970, there were few black pharmacists around, and they worked almost entirely in black communities. The Affirmative Action programs at universities such as Georgia and Mercer were intended to open previously locked doors to new careers and opportunities. After attending the lecture on pharmacy at the end of my junior year as an Animal Sciences major at Fort Valley, I decided pharmacy was the major for me.

I already had the prerequisites for a pharmacy

degree. I took courses in chemistry, organic, medicinal, and in the biological sciences such as anatomy and physiology, and also did some work in pharmacology, which studies the way drugs work in the body. The idea of a pharmacy degree was attractive not only in terms of the amount of time it would take me to complete it, but also in terms of having a career that would exercise my scientific skills. I'd become more confident about my aptitude for science studies, and wanted to put that confidence to work in a lucrative career.

Transferring to Mercer meant that I had to move up to Atlanta. I arranged to room with a family friend, and set about finding a trailer park where I could move my family. The first day of pharmacy school, I sat in the front row during orientation, where we were to hear the dean of the college, Dr. Littlejohn, tell us about a future in pharmacy. Part of Dean Littlejohn's speech included talking about how people should look in business, and he mentioned that men should have their hair cut close. "You must present yourselves in a professional manner, and that means looking professional," he declared. "You can't be professional when you've got hair up to the atmosphere looking like one of those drop-outs in San Francisco. No one's going to hire you looking like that."

There I was, sitting in the front row of the auditorium with my Afro, and wearing my bell-bottoms, looking nothing like what Dean Littlejohn said was "professional." I tried to keep quiet, but I just couldn't. "The length of a man's hair doesn't matter," I blurted out, my voice echoing off the auditorium's walls. The dean didn't know what to say, and before he could find any words, I continued. "Job performance and cleanliness do matter. If you discriminate based on hair, then you'll discriminate based on race. And you know, we have *got* to get past that."

After I said my piece, you could have heard a pin drop. I wasn't trying to be confrontational. I just had to say it. As with so many events in my life, when I saw that something had to be said or something had to be done, I said it or I did it. Doing nothing was never an option.

Dean Littlejohn did not respond, and as I left the auditorium, students stared at me. After that day, I was a known man on campus. I worked hard and got excellent grades, and soon became popular and respected among students and faculty alike. Before graduating, I became a member of Rho Chi, the national pharmacy honor society, which was indeed a real honor, since only those with excellent academic standing are invited to apply.

Two of my friends from Fort Valley, Johnny Early and Therman McKenzie, were also recruited with me the previous spring to the pharmacy program at Mercer, but they did not appear when the fall semester started. As a result, I was the sole black pharmacy student in my class. Not content with this situation, I returned to Fort Valley in the fall of 1970, along with the dean of the pharmacy college to recruit Johnny and Therman once again, and they began the program the following January. Eventually, by taking classes the following summer, they caught up with me, and the following fall we were altogether in the class scheduled for graduation in the spring of 1973.

Thanks to the Affirmative Action program, we continued actively recruiting qualified black students to the pharmacy program, and the classes behind ours ended up with eight black students—five more than ours. These students looked up to Therman, Johnny and me—the "first wave"—and actively supported and encouraged us as leaders of the black students at Mercer. We created the Black Student Pharmacy Association so we would have a place to meet and share ideas. Usually we got together once a month at my house.

As part of the pharmacy program, students worked at local hospitals. I was placed at DeKalb General Hospital working the 3-11 p.m. shift in the pharmacy. Our job was to help the pharmacist on duty prepare the medications, and then deliver them to the appropriate floor. DeKalb had a good pharmacy program, but it was clear from the beginning that the pharmacy was not embracing the Civil Rights Act. They had their quota: one black pharmacist and one technician, and they were not inclined to change those numbers significantly. Moreover, they were conservative. In both outward appearance and attitudes, the men were traditionalists. Their hair was closely cropped, while my Afro, a little bigger than when I first started college, stood out. They dressed in Oxford shirts, khaki pants and loafers, while I wore my favorite green bell-bottoms, shirts with sheen and platform shoes. It was no surprise that I was not readily accepted as a member of their clique. They spoke to me, but only when the topics of race and civil rights arose, as if those were the only things I could talk about.

"Say, Cornell," Jim Briscoe, the director of pharmacy, taunted me with a false smile as I loaded my cart for my rounds. "Are you one of them radicals? You know, are you one of them Communist Black Panthers?"

I always tried reason first. "Why do you think I might be a Communist or a Panther?"

He looked me up and down slowly. "It's obvious, isn't it?"

"Not to me," I replied firmly.

Needless to say, this and similar conversations always turned into heated debates, and I quickly earned a reputation for being "uppity," a denigrating term meant to keep you down and quiet—what anyone today would simply call "outspoken."

At first, I ignored the hushed conversation that abruptly stopped when I entered the room. I brushed off the comments about my appearance. I did my work, and I did it well. No one ever had to call Jim Briscoe to complain that I got an order wrong. My colleagues messed up orders all night long, but I was careful. I was thorough, efficient and professional. Nevertheless, Jim did not take to me. He was accustomed to black men who did as they were told, who were invisible, conformist men like the only black pharmacist at DeKalb, Al Richardson, who melt into the scenery and who cut his hair when he was told to. I was a product of my upbringing, experience, and I had a drive to be outstanding. As a result, I intimidated people like Briscoe. No matter how well I did my job, he would find some fault or other.

"Mac," Al told me urgently on more than one occasion, "you've got to stop having so much to say about everything."

I understood Al's position. He had a job to protect. I was young and fearless, and though I too had something important to protect, namely my family, I thought of my outspoken nature as an asset, not a liability.

"You get into these confrontations—"

"They're not confrontations," I interrupted. "They're discussions. I don't like confrontation, particularly."

He sighed. "You know they are not ready for you to have a voice."

"Maybe they aren't, but I am." Then I smiled. "And ready or not, here I come."

After a while, my resiliency wore thin. I dreaded 3 o'clock and the start of my eight-hour shift of unrelenting tension. Briscoe would fault me in ways that were too general for me to fix, or he would tell me to do something that was not required for me to fulfill my job description, like cut my hair. When I asked for clarification or refused an illegal order, he wrote me up as being "uncooperative."

I was at the top of my class at school, but at the bottom of the heap at work. Increasingly, I felt dehumanized by the atmosphere at DeKalb. All I wanted to do was work hard, learn and be respected as a human being. Without respect, the other elements of my experience were hollow.

I discussed with Harriet the prospect of quitting DeKalb. We needed the income to supplement my G.

I. funding, but I could find work at another hospital. As with all our other momentous decisions, Harriet was supportive.

Like my mother, Harriet is a wonderful listener. To this day, she is not the most expressive person in the world, and what she does express is typically the conclusion of an internal reasoning process that she keeps to herself. But those conclusions are golden, so when she has something to say, you would be advised to hear her out.

"If you've got to get out of there, then that's what you should do," she said one night in early spring of 1971. I had been working at DeKalb for about six months, and I had had it.

Having her consent lightened my burden considerably, but still, it was not an easy decision. When things weren't right, I looked to myself first, and asked whether or not I was at fault. Even though I had satisfied myself that I did everything I could do to make the job work, I wanted things to be different. Besides, I had finally gotten my family into brand-new public housing—a nice three-bedroom house for $67 a month—after another bitter experience with housing discrimination at a Douglasville trailer park, and I did not relish the prospect of having to move my family once again.

"If I resign next month, I could get the same job at another hospital before school lets out in June. That way I'd beat the rush," I said hopefully. Most students did not line up summer work before the academic year was over, so I knew that if I left DeKalb soon, I would be in a better position to find another, comparable position elsewhere.

Shortly thereafter, it was decided. I had just received my third evaluation, and it was not good. Of course, there was no specific criticism of my job performance, and so no real chance for me to correct whatever phantom errors I was making but Briscoe told me, "If you don't shape up by June, McBride, you're going to have to ship out."

"All right then," I responded noncommittally.

I set sail in April. The night I left DeKalb hospital for the last time, I was walking on air. It was a crisp, bright spring night, and I felt as though I was practically floating. My already happy mood brightened considerably as my 1964 Rambler American, which did not always start up right away, turned over like a dream. As I drove down Ponce de Leon Avenue, it was as if the whole world was opening up. I had left that job with my manhood and principles intact.

Chapter 9: Recognizing a Good Thing—A Really Good Thing

I went on to Grady Memorial Hospital, a predominantly black teaching hospital in the inner city that had opened originally in 1892 and was run by the city of Atlanta. There, I felt comfortable and respected. The white employees, by and large, did not display the same backward attitudes as those at DeKalb, and I quickly settled into my new routine.

That fall, at the start of my second year at Mercer in 1971, Therman and Johnny started at Grady, too. One day at work, Therman handed me a spray bottle.

"What's this?" I asked.

"For your 'fro," he responded with a wink, lightly tapping the side of his head. "It's the glycerin and water mix I told you I was using."

Therman had been using the mixture for a while, and I had commented on how good his hair was looking. He had agreed. "I'll bring you some of what I'm trying," he had told me. "But don't get your hopes up," he joked. "I don't know if you'll look as good as me."

Therman was a handsome guy, a sturdy five feet eleven and about 190 pounds. He was a farm boy from an old black Georgia farm family, born and bred, up at 5 every morning to tend to the pigs and cows. He knew how to work hard and then leave that work when it was done and go have a good time. Popular at school, Therman was a member of a fraternity, liked to party like any other college-age guy and fit in seamlessly at school. He was not confrontational or particularly outspoken, but he was studious. And always generous, Therman shared the mixture with some other guys, and was happy to let me try it, too.

I had complained to Therman about my own paltry Afro on a number of occasions. It just did not want to grow the way other guys' did, because it was still too hard, which meant the ends broke easily. Harriet would braid my hair nightly, and then I'd pick it out in the morning to make it stand up, but still I just could not get it big.

He handed the bottle to me. "All right," I nodded, eager to try something new. I took the bottle. "I'll try anything right about now."

"Good. The ladies like it, too. Oh, wait. I forgot you're a married man!"

"Yes, I am. And my wife has excellent taste. When you are as mature as I am," I said, ribbing him over our six-year age difference, "you will understand how important that is."

"All right, all right," he laughed. "I think you'll like this spray. It's good stuff."

He was right. It *was* good. Right away, my hair softened up, and my Afro was more manageable. But I
could tell straightaway that it could be better. I also
knew that there were no hair care products on the market formulated specifically for hard, brittle hair.
Nothing made hair soft, which was exactly what people like me needed if we wanted to have decent Afros.
There were products for men, Easy Comb and Oil
Sheen, however these products undermined hair
health. Easy Comb and Oil Sheen were used in tan-
dem: Easy Comb allowed you to comb your hair, but
made it hard and brittle afterwards, which my hair
already was and just the opposite of what I needed. Oil
Sheen was meant to be sprayed on for shine after you
combed your hair out, but it just made hair look oily.
Neither product, as those of us who used them knew,
was any good for developing a healthy Afro. There
were pomades, too, but those did not work on Afros.
Instead, like Oil Sheen, those products simply made
hair greasy and limp. The formula Therman gave me,
though not perfect, accomplished in one treatment
what Easy Comb and Oil Sheen did not accomplish in
two. There was also Johnson Products, which put out
Ultra and Afro sheen, and Pro Line out in California
had some products, but otherwise, the male hair-care
category was sorely wanting. Moreover, neither
Johnson nor Pro Line had developed anything much
better than Easy Comb and Oil Sheen.

    Afros were so popular by the early '70s among
black men and women, it was actually surprising that
no company had developed a product to soften the

Afro. Before, men had kept their hair short and used pomades for shine and waves, so there was not any call for products to make men's hair soft. The Black Power movement that began in the '60s affected hairstyles, and James Brown's "Black and Proud" helped inspire the popularity of the Afro. The more I thought about it, and the more I used the glycerin and water solution, the more surprised I was. Maybe we need to do something about that, I said to myself.

Within weeks I noticed even more improvement in the softness and comb-ability of my hair. The only drawback was that it looked like water droplets on the hair unless massaged in thoroughly. It wasn't as bad as the other products, but it could have been better. In its current form, I was not satisfied with it. So, I decided to perfect the formula. It was as if I knew immediately that, if done right, the formula could fill a current need.

Not only was there a desire for a good product, but also I had the desire to put my creative talents to work. Experimenting with formulas was a great outlet for those talents. I loved the process of solving problems, of making something good even better, and finding out how my ideas could positively affect others. It was like when I ran my own janitorial business while an airman, where I implemented innovative changes to the way the Air Force readied houses for new tenants. With the hair formula experimentations, I was looking to be innovative in an area of the hair-care industry that was sorely lacking for new ideas.

One of my professors, Dr. Frankie, ended up giving

me some good, and needed, advice that helped me figure out a formula that would soften and strengthen
hair without drowning it in oil.

While I was working in the school lab one day, he
walked in. "You are looking serious, Cornell," he said.

"I am, Dr. Frankie," I replied, shaking my head in
frustration. I told him about the mixture beading up
on hair. "It mixes well in the bottle, but once it's on…"
I shrugged, out of ideas. "It needs *something*."

"Try some sodium laurel sulfate. That ought to
help."

"About how much?"

"Try .1 percent."

I was grateful for the advice. Though I was an outspoken person since childhood, I was never one to
ignore advice. If someone had something to say, I was
ready to hear it. If one brain working on a problem
was good, then two should be better.

After experimenting to find the right mixture of
ingredients, I hit upon the right recipe. Next, I took my
new formula over to Grady and made up some batch-
es in their lab. Then I started handing out bottles to
folks at the hospital and to fellow students on campus.
Within days, people were coming back for more. It
worked as well on their hair as it had on mine, making
it cottony soft.

"Therman," I said excitedly one day at work, "this
could be big. *Really* big." We were taking inventory in
the pharmacy's cavernous storeroom. "I finally got the
formula right. Man, I'm telling you, I have to beat people away if I don't have their product when they come
looking for it!"

"What, that water and glycerin I gave you?" he asked absentmindedly, not looking up from his clipboard. "Anyone can do that, Mac."

"I know, I know," I responded, beaming. "But it's not just glycerin and water anymore. I've got the formula down. We've got to go into business, I'm telling you. This is an *untapped* market."

Therman was not initially impressed. I knew I had to persuade him.

"Think about it. How long have folks been trying to straighten their hair? Ever since technology gave them the means to do it, black people have been trying to change their hair, to straighten it out. But now, look around. What do you see? Afros everywhere. *Afros.* Naturally black hair! But no one's helping us grow it. No one's helping us keep it healthy." I raised my eyebrows. "But *we* can help them keep it healthy. You know we couldn't give it away fast enough– even before I changed the formula. People can't get enough. For the first time, black men can soften their hair, and it grows. I'm proud of that, aren't you?"

Therman shook his head, intrigued, but still uncertain. "How are we going to start a business? We're in *college*, Mac. We don't even graduate for another year. And what about money? We don't have any extra, let alone any kind of start-up money. And where are we going to get the supplies? The right chemicals and bottles? And then, even if we do, how are we going to get this stuff into the store? Besides, I'm still thinking about dental school." He had been talking for some time about becoming a dentist once finishing his college work.

"Therman, we cannot wait to do this. Someone else is going to get to it if we don't, because almost every black man I know wears an Afro today. Remember when the Commodores used to play Fort Valley? Have you seen Lionel Ritchie's 'fro lately?" The Commodores had become a big group since they started as students at Tuskegee University. They were playing all over the country by the time Therman handed me the hair solution, and they would soon become one of the best-known bands in the world. "You know he is not the only one. "

Suddenly, the door swung open. "McBride!" a voice bellowed.

We turned toward the voice, and saw an imposing hulk of a man standing at the entrance of the storeroom.

"Yeah," I said, annoyed at being interrupted. Who was this guy interrupting my business planning?

"I hear you've got a product." The man stepped forward eagerly. "See?" he said, pulling a pick comb from the top of his head. There were a lot of hairs on it. "I grew it out, but it got to this length and now it just breaks off."

I looked at Therman knowingly. Then I pulled a pick out of my pocket and ran it through my own hair. "I used to have that, too. But now look." I held out the pick for him to see. It was clean.

"Mmm," his voice rumbled deep in his throat. "How much a bottle?"

"Tell you what," I said, putting my hand on his shoulder. "I'm still working out the pricing, so let me give you a bottle to try, and then the next one I'll be ready to sell. Okay?"

I steered him toward the storeroom door. As we walked out, the man stopped suddenly and said, "Oh, hey. Earlene said to tell you that you'd best not be giving me any product before she gets hers. She said don't forget she asked you this morning, and you promised her something this afternoon."

Looking back over my shoulder at Therman, I said, "Oh, tell Earlene not to worry. I said 3 o'clock and I meant it."

When I returned to the storeroom, Therman was ready to go into business. "Cornell, we have got to talk to Johnny." "Dental school? What dental school?" his expression seemed to say.

Therman was a smart man, and he knew a good idea when he saw it. I knew I couldn't start a business without him. After all, it was Therman who brought the initial formula to me, and in doing so, got things started. And not only that, in those days, we were like two peas in a pod. Along with Johnny Early, Therman and I did everything together. It would not be right pursuing a brand-new, and potentially lucrative venture, unless we did it together.

"Well," I smiled. "Let's do it." I tapped my wristwatch. "Time's a wasting." And with that, we backed right into the beginning of what would become a multimillion-dollar hair-care corporation.

Chapter 10: Introducing M&M Products Company

Everything about the company that became M&M Products, and I mean everything, we learned and built from scratch. Starting out, the only things we had were a product and small customer base. The list of what we did not have was much, much longer: a manufacturing facility, enough ingredient or bottle supplies to get started properly, a product name, company name, a logo, or even the seed money to buy or develop these things. We were not equipped to manufacture and distribute large quantities to that base. After all, I had been working out of one of the Grady labs, producing only enough product to fill about a dozen or so bottles at a time.

There were other initial obstacles to overcome. We had to learn about FDA requirements for manufacturing products, meet with suppliers to price stocks of ingredients and spray bottles, consult with graphic designers about the product name and logo design and process of silk screening it onto the bottle—once we got around to figuring out what they would be—as well as learn that the label had to be flame treated onto the bottle so that any spilling of the product onto the outside would not make the label smear off. We also had to fill out and submit the necessary paperwork for starting a joint company, determine if we could locate an affordable and suitable manufacturing facility, and find the time to continue with a full-time course schedule."Mixing medications or mixing hair formulas," I held up my palms, and smiled. "Mixing is mixing."

"No, you know what I mean. We're *practitioners.* Besides, I'm thinking of going to grad school. I want my Ph.D. in Pharmacology." He was considering the graduate program in Pharmacology at Purdue, a prestigious program at a prestigious school. I did not blame him for feeling pulled in that direction. It was important to Johnny to do something with his life that would have a positive impact on others.

He was, by nature, a quiet, contemplative guy, but when he spoke, he had something important to say. At five feet seven and 140 pounds, Johnny was not a big man, but he was a big thinker and an exceptional student. What he lacked in physical bulk, he more than made up for in intellectual power. Johnny was an intellectual radical. In this respect he was the complete opposite of the more socially conformist, Therman. He wrote articles for national magazines, organized the national pharmaceutical college studies group, and, from his vantage point at Mercer University, had a lot to say about how life was for black students looking to break into historically white careers. Like Therman, however, students and faculty alike respected Johnny. He was a good friend, and a good person to go into business with.

I leaned forward in my chair. "Johnny, this is an opportunity. Nobody else is doing this. And I'm telling you, M.E.M. is going to be *big*."

"'M.E.M.'?" he asked quizzically.

"McKenzie, Early, McBride. Or McBride, Early, McKenzie. See, either way, you're right in the middle of it." At least the company name was now one item checked off on our list. I had also done my homework by the time Therman and I sat down to pitch the idea to Johnny.

"It's a big undertaking," he said hesitantly.

"We can do it. One step at a time."

"Mac's run a business before," Therman reassured him. "We won't need to sweat the small stuff."

I threw everything I had at him. If I gave him a chance to think about it, I knew we would lose him to graduate school. "The paperwork is a formality. We need a name for the product—something catchy that tells the buyer exactly what they're getting—and then we are good to go. We just have to make the time to create the product and then canvas the salons and stores. Right now, we have to market it; we have to get it on the shelves ourselves. The product will sell itself once people try it, but we've got to get it into their hands, first. You've seen how popular it is here at school, and at Grady."

It was true. Johnny and I sometimes worked the same shift at Grady Hospital, where I made up the product on breaks between filling prescriptions, making medications and taking inventory in the vast pharmacy stock room—there were no computer-based inventories in those days. He knew the Mercer and

Grady communities were microcosms of any other community you could find in the South, and in my work I had access to most of the hospital departments and their staff. The people who clamored for our hair-softening product at school and the hospital would be no different from any other folks who were looking to improve their hair quality.

"Besides, you can always go to grad school," I repeated the line I used on Therman. "Now's the time to start a business."

"Let me think about it," Johnny offered. True to his word, he did give the proposal serious consideration, but in the end, he said, "Fellas, I'm choosing Purdue."

Therman and I decided to move forward anyway, now as M&M Products. Though we were disappointed not to have Johnny with us, we knew he would go on to become a successful scientist, and we were as happy for him in his choice as he became for us in ours.

We still had to come up with the all-important product name. One day, back once again at Mercer's student center, we brainstormed.

"The name's got to say what it does," I started.

"It makes your 'fro soft," Therman offered.

"Right, and it *keeps* it soft."

"Mm-hmm, it stays soft," Therman continued, thinking out loud.

We thought about it for a moment more, then almost simultaneously, we called out, "stay soft 'fro!"

And in that eureka moment, Sta Sof Fro was born. Now we needed to settle on a design for the product name and find start-up money. Being college students and, in my case, also a family man, it was not as if we had any extra cash lying around, but I managed to pull together $250. Therman found a banker at C&S Bank, who was also an alumnus of Mercer, and through him Therman secured a $250 loan for start-up costs. With $500, M&M Products was in business. With that initial investment, we would produce our first 1,000 bottles of Sta Sof Fro.

After that, things began moving fast—so fast, in fact, that from the time we started M&M, and even after the company reached its peak in the mid-1980s, we never stopped to get our bearings. We were on a fast ride, and there was no time to slow down. If either one of us had wanted off it, we would have to have jumped.

We had our product formula, product and company names, and now, with the money in place, we were ready to figure out more of the details of the Sta Sof Fro bottle's look. Everything that the product did, along with who M&M was, had to be on that bottle. This product was formulated for a specific market and demographic—there wouldn't be any crossover to the white or straight hair market, and it seemed clear to me that our customers needed to know who was making the product specifically for them. "It's important we use our identity as black professionals," I said. "People are going to buy this product without knowing anything about us. We've got to make the product tell them." So we did. "Developed by Black Pharmacists for Their own Hair" was printed on the back of every bottle.

We told a white pharmacist at Grady Hospital that we were going into business for ourselves, and he

enthusiastically offered to draw up a logo for the bottle. "I'm a cartoonist, too," he told us. Within seconds,
he drew up two sketches, a male Afro and female Afro.
Though the product was intended initially for men
because of the dearth of black male hair-care products,
plenty of women were wearing Afros, too, and we did
not want to leave out another potential goldmine.

We also solicited help from Annie Washington,
who was herself a graduate of Mercer's School of
Pharmacy, and who worked in administration while
Therman and I were students at Mercer. Annie's
administrative and creative assistance was invaluable.
It was she who wrote the copy for the back panel of the
bottle.

We next found a silk-screening company, Nash
Screen Printing Company, housed in an old, run-down
building. We were a little apprehensive. When we
went inside, we were met by the proprietor, a little old
white lady who looked more suitable for sitting on a
rocker with her knitting than the labor of silk- screening and flame-treating labels. She surprised us, both in
her estimate of what it would cost for our inventory
and the quality of the resulting job. We used Nash
Screen Printing Company for years afterward, and
eventually bought it.

With all the product and company details complete,
all we had to do was make our first thousand bottles.
But there was one significant problem, and for a brief
while, it seemed insurmountable: manufacturing
space. Leasing a facility was far too expensive. At the
same time, we were about to graduate, and that meant
we were about to leave our jobs at Grady—which

meant leaving Grady's lab. Besides, we could not run a business, however small, out of the hospital. For a while, planning ground to a halt. We worried that we would be finished before we even got started. Then Therman hit upon a brilliant solution. "We can use space in the basement of my house," he told me. After scouting it, we decided it would work for the moment. Though small and not a site at which we could expand with the growth of the business, it was big enough, and we could have it cheap. We also found out that the FDA only required a clean facility for production, and once it was inspected, we were in business.

We had our thousand bottles silk-screened with the product's name, Sta Sof Fro on the front in bold black letters, which contrasted well with the white bottle. On the back of the bottle were our company name, location and our slogan. In the early 1970s, there was no governmental oversight of products such as ours that required companies to list the formulas, and we saw no reason to disclose the contents, especially since we were not able to patent our formula.

We had tried to patent it, knowing that, if we grew by leaps and bounds as we expected to, eventually the big hair-care companies were going to take notice of our product, and they would certainly try to enter into the market. Even if we grew quickly, we would never be able to compete with the size of established companies like Johnson Products, the premier black-owned hair-care company, so we wanted the protection of a patent on the formula for Sta Sof Fro. We consulted an attorney but were told we did not have a patentable product.

"You can trademark the name," the attorney told Therman and me. "And you should do that. But you can't do anything with the formula."

"But why not?" Therman asked.

"Yeah," I chimed in. "Why not? No one else—and I mean *no other company* is making a product like this. I guarantee you that. Can't we protect it? It *is* original."

"It's the ingredients, the chemistry. The formula itself just is not original. Besides, even with a patented formula people can get around them and come close to the original. You really can't secure your product the way you want to, though I understand the impulse. Sorry."

That struck us as peculiar, but Therman and I both agreed that the attorney must know more than we did about it, so we let it go. Later on, we would regret not pursuing the patent more vigorously. For a couple of years after Sta Sof Fro started taking off, it was considered a revolutionary miracle formula because no one knew its contents. Initially, with no big company interested enough in analyzing the contents—a process that requires significant physical and financial resources—not having the formula listed on the bottle was a lifesaver for our little company. But once the government legislated ingredients be listed, and larger companies began to take notice of our near monopoly on the hair-softening market, we had the competition's scalding hot breath at the backs of our necks, and it would prove difficult competing against much larger outfits while we were still so young.

Though we were thorough in our research, we had much to learn, and that included seeking more than

one expert opinion when it came to important decisions such as patents. At least we did go forward with
copywriting Sta Sof Fro, and set ourselves up as officers of our company. After consulting with a lawyer,
Therman insisted I be named president of M&M
because of my previous business experience, so I was
effectively the face of the company. Therman became
the executive treasurer and vice president, but we set
things up so that we were equal partners in every
aspect of M&M. I had no desire to be autocratic just
because of my title. We had always consulted with
each other about everything, and there would be no
difference now.

Though I had always been involved in side-busi-
nesses in addition to whatever I was doing, whether it
was collecting scrap metal as a kid, landscaping, trying to get into raising hogs and turkeys, or creating a
janitorial business while in the Air Force, this new venture with Therman did not feel like anything on the
side. It quickly became the focus of our attention. Just
as quickly, we were outgrowing Therman's basement.
In addition, we were both mere weeks away from
graduating from Mercer University with our Bachelor
of Science degrees in Pharmacy—and I was about to
become a father for a third time!

Chapter 11: Some Things in Life Are Really Free

Therman, Johnny and I graduated from Mercer College in June of 1973. Upon graduating, Johnny prepared for Emory's graduate pharmacology program. Therman and I went straight to work at Revco Pharmacy. Because M&M was just getting started, we needed the stability of day jobs. I knew, however, that there was not a lot of upward mobility in working for a corporate pharmacy. Initially, I had considered opening up my own pharmacy in Savannah—I even had the location scouted—but the security of the Revco position allowed me to focus much of my M&M attention on developing a client-base for Sta Sof Fro.

There was just one problem. We had no idea how to price our product. When I ran my janitorial business, I could base pricing on the hours it took to clean a house, plus the cost of cleaning supplies. With Sta Sof Fro, we knew how much the supplies cost, and we also knew the retail cost of various hair-care products, but we did not know what the retail mark-up was.

Moreover, since there really was no other comparable product out there, Sta Sof Fro was unique. We had no idea how to quantify that uniqueness.

"We need a distributor," Therman said. "Say we sell to him for $20 a case. That's $1.65 a bottle for a case of 12. He can turn around and sell the case for $30, and make $10 a case."

"Sounds good," I agreed. "Let's talk to Roscoe."

We sought out Roscoe White, one of the best rack jobbers in Atlanta, who we knew through Revco. He was the distributor for some products sold at Revco, and was a guy who had been around the block more than once. So, we called him up to see about having him be our guy for distribution.

"Come on over," he said over the phone. "But make it early. I've got a lot of stops to make."

We headed over to Roscoe's house to make a presentation of our product, hoping he would take us on as our distributor. First, however, he set us straight about pricing. Therman and I were like two eager boys thinking about how much we could make without knowing the first thing about how the system worked.

Roscoe, on the other hand, knew how things worked, and if he thought he could make a dollar with our product, his help would be invaluable. In fact, he would prove instrumental in getting Sta Sof Fro established throughout Atlanta. The meeting turned out to be revelatory, as we had no clue how the distributor-retailer system worked.

After sitting through our presentation, he got down to business. "It's like this," he said, his large frame taking up the entirety of his living room chair.

Therman and I sat gingerly on the edge of the sofa across from him. "You've got your pricing for selling to the store direct, and your pricing for selling to a distributor, namely me."

We nodded in acknowledgment, and he continued with his lesson. "Say Sta Sof Fro is retailing at $2.50. Now, that's about a dollar more than other products of its kind, but as you yourself said earlier, those products are only cousins. There's nothing else out there like Sta Sof Fro. Okay, so now you want to know how to price it once you bring in a distributor."

"Exactly," I said. "Everybody's got to win in this venture, not just us, or you, or the store. And the customer has got to feel like they're getting their money's worth."

"True," Roscoe agreed. "So here's what you've got to do. You sell to me. Then I sell to the retailer so that I make a profit, and then the retailer sells to the customer to make a profit."

Therman and I nodded, completely absorbed in learning this part of business that was entirely new to us.

"To get you started with me, I buy at $13.33 a dozen. Then I'm going to sell to the stores at $18 or $20 a dozen. Retailer makes the most money, by the way. That's just the way it works."

We found out that, normally, a distributor does not want to pay a third and a third for a brand-new product. Instead, most distributors did a third and 40. But Roscoe cut us a break.

And with that, we had ourselves an official distributor for Sta Sof Fro. If things were moving swiftly beforehand, when Roscoe came on the scene, we hit the rapids. Therman and I did not, however, simply rely on Roscoe to get our product out there.

Every day of the week, Therman or I went door to door at salons, beauty supply stores and barber shops to sell Sta Sof Fro—anywhere where there was a decision-maker, someone who could, on the spot, decide to put our product on the shelf. I enjoyed meeting new people and talking to them about the product. Even that early in the life of the company, I knew that I would learn a lot about what worked and what did not work with a product by having my ear to the ground. Knowing what people who used the product thought, from stylists to customers, would help us sell it. Not only that, as a naturally gregarious person, I connected well with customers and the stores that stocked Sta Sof Fro.

I am sure that one of the main reasons for the groundswell of popularity enjoyed by Sta Sof Fro was our practice of heavy sampling. We always had a plan to get the product on the shelves, and that plan almost always included sampling. The reason was simple: once we got the product into a person's hands, we knew that person would be back for more. So, sampling was crucial when we could not get Sta Sof Fro on the shelves at a store.

"Good morning!" I boomed to a salesgirl as Therman and I strode through the doors at a local drug store. "Can we speak to your buying manager?" Dressed in nice suits, and carrying a box of Sta Sof Fro, we had an air about us of successful businessmen.

"All right," she said, a little startled. "That's Mr. Walker. I'll get him," and she disappeared to the back of the store.

A short while later, a balding heavyset white man ambled out. "Hey," he said, his hands shoved deep into his pants pockets. "What can I do for you boys today?"

I cringed inside, as I am sure Therman did, but I kept smiling. "Hello, sir. Mr. Walker, how are you today? My name is Cornell McBride, and this is my business partner, Therman McKenzie." Therman stretched out his right hand, and the store manager reluctantly took it. "We operate M&M Products Company," I continued. "And we have formulated a hair-care product specially for Afros." I pointed at my head. "This product is revolutionary, and I am sure your black customers would buy out your supply."

Therman handed over a bottle, and the manager scrutinized it skeptically. "I don't know," he said handing the bottle back. "I don't have much call for this 'Afro' hair stuff."

"No, no," Therman said, waving the bottle back to him. "You keep it. In fact, we've got a dozen bottles right here, that we can leave on consignment."

"Consignment?"

"Right," Therman continued. "No cost to you. Just a little shelf space. We'll come by next week to see how it's doing."

Walker breathed in deeply, as though he was giving the prospect great consideration. Then he said. "All right. Consignment. But just for a week. Y'all come back and take it away when it doesn't move."

"Oh, it will move," I assured him. "Just tell us where to put it and we'll even stock it ourselves."

He walked us over to the "Ethnic" section of the store, and pointed to an empty shelf at eye-level. "You can have that one there." Then he shuffled away.

Once we put our 12 bottles up neatly on the shelf, we went outside to my car, where we got another box of product. Then we stood outside the store and started handing out free samples to men walking by. "Give it a try," we said enthusiastically. "It will do wonders for your hair's quality." "Now, you look like a man who knows how to care for your hair. That is one impressive Afro! Want to make it even more impressive?" "You, sir, do not have to live with a paltry Afro, no sir! Try this." "Yes, it's a free sample." "Now, when you find it's working, just step inside this store here. The shelf is stocked with plenty of Sta Sof Fro. And if it's out, you ask for Mr. Walker. You let him know you want your Sta Sof Fro, and we'll make sure more gets on the shelf." It was a wonder we did not lose our voices with all that talking.

We sampled our product until we had none left, and then went on to the next place. Others declined to stock Sta Sof Fro, albeit in a more congenial manner than Mr. Walker, and we offered the same consignment deal. Then we stood outside the store and gave out samples there.

The more samples we gave out, the more sales we made by the end of the month. Mitchell Brothers alone, for example, sold 12 dozen bottles of Sta Sof Fro in a single week. We were hot in Atlanta, and for almost a year, we did not try to venture beyond the city. Because we were so hands-on and because we were certainly doing well in Atlanta, and there was still plenty to learn about saturating the market in our hometown. Atlanta became "our own little United

States." That's what a distributor told us we should do. We knew him from Revco, where he distributed LeConte Products. "If I were you," he told us one time, "I would stay right here in Atlanta, and make it your own little United States. If you can't sell it here, it won't sell."

He was right. There were benefits to remaining in Atlanta, not the least of which was that we saved on expenses we would have incurred if we immediately tried to go regional. So, we followed his wise advice, and it worked.

When we returned to Mr. Walker's store, he was just a bit friendlier, and put in a substantial order to stock several shelves. Soon enough, Sta Sof Fro was not simply stocked on shelves at drug stores and salons, it was prominently displayed and, because of its effectiveness, it kept its prominence. This happened at every store where we placed Sta Sof Fro on consignment. People tried it and then went into those stores and asked for more. Invariably, the buyers were very happy to see us when we came back to check on how the product was selling.

Sta Sof Fro was not just a solid product, it was a product with actual people from the community behind it. Not only that, but early on, we did not have market research—data that told us who was buying what, when, where and how often. Instead, we learned that by keeping our ears to the ground and paying attention to what we heard. Later, I kept up the practice of visiting. Oftentimes, I would go out into the field without any idea in mind other than to say hello.

But I also got information that, had I waited instead for the market research data to come back, would have put us a year behind the times.

Between manufacturing, packaging, sampling, pounding the pavement to find stores that would carry our product, and working full time at Revco, Therman and I barely had time to breathe. Within months of officially putting out Sta Sof Fro, we were having trouble keeping up with demand—even with Roscoe's great distribution network. We needed more help.

"Why don't we call Roosevelt Johnson?" I suggested to Therman. "You remember him from Fort Valley."

"Oh, yeah. Sure, I remember him."

My instinct was, and still is, to look to my community for help. When I had any sort of success, I wanted to share that with people I knew. Sometimes that was a positive thing, and sometimes not. But it was important to me to lift up people I knew who needed a chance.

"He was always an ambitious guy. Always wanted to get into business," I said.

"Personable, too," Therman continued. "He always talked a good talk."

Indeed, Roosevelt was a perfect fit. He was a natural salesman, and Sta Sof Fro being a quality product only enhanced that native ability. We called him, and he was interested.

Because we were still just starting out, we knew Roosevelt would be taking a risk coming to work with us. He had just married his college sweetheart, Sarah Green, and we knew how hard it was to start a life together on a venture not guaranteed to succeed. So, we promised him a percentage of the company once it got off the ground. Things started off well. Roosevelt was, indeed, a natural. Within a few months, however, things changed for him.

"Sarah's pregnant," he told us with a mixture of excitement, pride and nervousness.

"That's wonderful news, Roose!" Therman and I congratulated him.

"The thing is," he hesitated. "I think we need stability. You know, for the family and all."

Of course we understood. We were sad to lose him, but did not begrudge him the safety of a company job and steady paycheck. Eventually, as it turned out, Roosevelt became a preacher and now lives in Savannah.

We had some important decisions to make. Demand was high, and we worried about inventory getting too low because there were not enough hours in the day to work as full-time pharmacists and produce Sta Sof Fro. Somehow, M&M had to expand. We knew we needed more room for production, but we had other questions to consider. Should we hire someone to help with manufacturing? Should we quit Revco and devote ourselves completely to M&M Products? In the end, we decided to stay at Revco at least a little while longer, but find a bigger production facility in order to meet the demand for Sta Sof Fro.

Chapter 12: Moving Up

"Let's re-invest our profits," I said to Therman. It was a Saturday morning, I think, about six months into our new venture. We were in our "production facility" in Therman's basement, where it was cold and dreary, having a meeting about keeping up with customer demand for Sta Sof Fro. It had been raining for the past few days, and I was ready to see some sunshine. We were tired, too, working seven days a week. I missed my family—our newborn, Sholanda, was too charming to be away from so much, and my older kids, Sheila and Cornell Jr. , needed their dad's attention just as much as Sta Sof Fro did. Then there was the ever-present promise I had kept close to my heart since I was 10 years old. I still had that house to build for my mother. So I said to Therman, "We need to expand. We're turning out inventory so fast we can hardly keep up. The way to keep up and expand that is re-invest what we've made."

We were making enough off of our small operation to be able to pay ourselves a small salary plus put money back into the company for supplies. Things were going so well that we had not even begun advertising the product yet. Instead, our initial success was due to word of mouth and pounding the pavement. I made a gut estimation, based on the return business and positive comments, that we had an 80% acceptance rate from our door-to-door sales alone—and just like at Mercer and Grady, people kept coming back for more. Not only were we gaining customers, but also the existing ones were already becoming loyal to the product.

"That's a good idea," Therman agreed, "but we don't have enough right now to rent a quality facility."

"I'm thinking of buying," I responded.

"What! We can't do that. How are we going to get that kind of loan?"

"Now, hold on. Harriet and I have been thinking about buying a home. What if we get one with a basement that's bigger than this shoebox?"

Therman considered my suggestion. "Right, right. Then we can save on rent and put profits right back into the company."

"And," I said with growing excitement, "when it's time to expand again, we'll have the money for a major manufacturing facility—or at least the foundation for a decent-sized loan."

With that, Harriet and I began searching for a suitable home. I was proud, and Harriet beamed as she moved from room to room at each house we viewed.

After looking at quite a few houses in our price range, we found one that would suit both our personal and career needs. It was a tidy two-bedroom, brick house with brand-new carpeting, a den we could turn

into a nursery for Sholanda, awnings over the windows and a car park. Although it was just miles from
the projects where we had been living, it was worlds
away. Built on the edge of a golf course in the '50s in
southeast Atlanta, along with the other homes in the
neighborhood, it was a suburban community made for
young families on their way up. Though originally a
white neighborhood, black homeowners increasingly
populated it, and Harriet and I added to that number.
For $22,000, it was a good buy. Harriet and I discussed
once more what life would be like with a home-based
business.

"I do not plan for the business to stay here forever,"
I told her. "It is going to take off, I am sure of that. But
we're not ready to take the next step to trying to buy
or lease a facility."

Several weeks later, we found a home, and about a
month after that, it was ours. "The real estate agent
called," Harriet said matter-of-factly one day when I
arrived home from the pharmacy. "We just closed on
the house." A small smile danced across her lips.

"Yes!" I exclaimed, and swept her up into my arms.
We had scrimped and saved every last penny, and now
it was paying off. We were property owners—and
there was a big basement for us to use as headquarters
for M&M product manufacturing.

"We can help out, the kids and I," Harriet offered
after I set her back down on her own feet. "We always
talk about teaching them how a business runs. We can
help put the product together." In those days, Harriet
was not particularly confident, except when it came to
her home and children. She was uncompromising

about their care and education, which in this case included having them help with the new business.

I smiled, suddenly remembering the house down on Gordon Road and my father's liquor house. "Remember I told you about that?" I said to Harriet.

"Mm-hmm," she nodded.

I shook my head. "He had a knack, that's for sure. If only he abstained from consuming his own inventory!" I thought about our elder children learning, from the ground up, how a solid business begins. "You're right. This will be good for them."

Every inch of the basement was taken up with M&M-related materials. There was enough room to set up a decently sized assembly line. We had our boxed supply of Sta Sof Fro-labeled bottles on one side, along with separate boxes of spray bottle tops. Lined up next to those were the supplies of ingredients, which were kept separately in large containers. On the other side of the basement were cardboard boxes stacked flat and ready to be put together. In those we put 12-count bottles of the finished product and then sealed for delivery to our various outlets and individual customers. Across the length of the basement we set up tables on which we assembled the elements once Therman or I had mixed together the recipe.

Sheila and Cornell Jr. enthusiastically took up their parts of the assembly process. Working on the miniature assembly line became part of their daily chores, and they could not go out to play before they poured and packed enough product to keep up the inventory. Standing on either side of the table, usually next to their mother, they poured the product into bottles, twisted on the spray tops, and then neatly placed each bottle in a box. Then Cornell Jr. taped the box up with heavy-duty tape, and Sheila labeled the box with the name of its destination. More than once I glanced over at my family with pride and gratitude as we all worked together to put out Sta Sof Fro. It wasn't long before we were putting out larger and larger quantities of inventory.

It was exciting to be part of this new adventure. We were turning out inventory so fast, and our revenue increased dramatically. One night, as Harriet and I were getting ready for bed, I pulled out a large roll of bills and placed it on the dresser along with my keys, watch and a few other sundries.

As I crawled into bed, Harriet asked for some cash. "Cornell Jr. needs new shoes," she said.

I smiled wearily, pleased to be going to sleep after a long day of work, with my family tucked safely in for the night. "He never stops moving, does he."

"No, he does not. I'm going to the store tomorrow. Let me take some of that cash on the dresser."

"Nuh-uh," I muttered, and turned over. "Not that."

"What? Why?" she demanded. "There's cash right there. Your son needs new shoes. What more is there to know?"

Harriet's dander was rarely raised, but when it was, watch out—especially when it came to her children. The otherwise quiet and laconic Harriet could be a lioness if she had to.

I reached over to pat her hand. "I will get you the money, okay? But not that money over there. That's not mine."

"Not yours?" she asked, in disbelief. "Then whose is it?"

"It belongs to the business. It's M&M's money."

"And just *who* is M&M if it's not you and Therman?"

I could not help but laugh a little, even though I knew that would make her even madder. "M&M is the company I *work for*. I get paid by the company, but that over there is M&M's profits. I have to take that money and deposit it into M&M's account. That money goes to supplies and so forth. I have to keep track of it otherwise this business is not going to last."

Harriet was not interested in why she could not use some of that money for her family. It seemed clear to her that there was a direct line between me, the work performed to generate that money, and what was sitting right there on the dresser. I realized that we never really had that kind of money lying around the house before. M&M was pulling in a lot, and that day I just did not have time to go to the bank to deposit it, as I usually did. I do not think Harriet had ever encountered quantity like that. When we were in Plattsburgh, I handled all the money from the janitorial business, which in any case was not nearly the amount I was earning from M&M. It's sort of like how people are today with credit cards. We tend not to connect the credit card with actual money that we will have to pay eventually, just like I realized it was hard for Harriet to connect the cash on the dresser with a formal company to whom that cash belonged. If she used it, we'd still have to pay it back at some point.

I realized then how important it is to think about

your own business. It was not like Harriet did not understand numbers and money. She was an expert at stretching a dollar, had been intimately involved with the Plattsburgh planning and budgeting that had got us to where we were now, and is today an intuitively excellent investor. But before M&M, we always had only our personal money, and the money on the dresser was company funds. Though I was learning as I went with this new business, my previous experience and natural instincts were helping me to understand a fundamental rule of business: always make sure you keep track of every penny.

I held out, not giving her any of the money sitting on the dresser. But first thing in the morning, I made sure she had what she needed to get Cornell Jr. his new shoes.

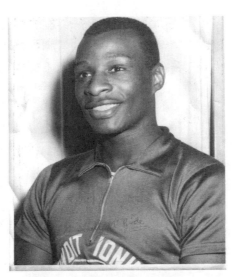

20 Year Old Cornell McBride Sr. in
The United States Air Force

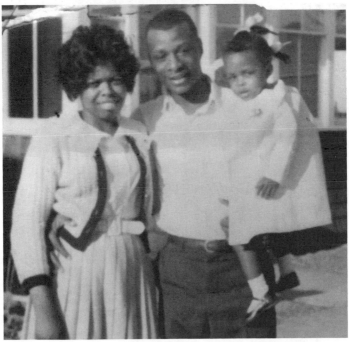

Harriet, Cornell, and Sheila McBride in Plattsburgh New York

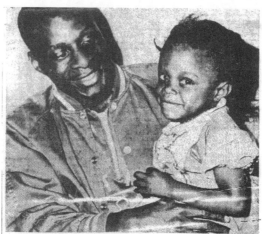

FINDS IT ROUGH — Cornell McBride plays with his daughter, Sheila, 2. McBride claims he spent more than a year looking for an apartment in and around the city of Plattsburgh. Once his family had to live in a roached-infested tenement with no bathing facilities. Do the landlords here hate Negroes? "I don't know," he said. "Some of them tried to be nice when they told me their apartments were rented. But their ads stayed in the paper for weeks afterward." (P-R Photo by Kathy Brothers)

Sheila and Cornell Sr. in Plattsburgh Press Republican News Paper in 1965

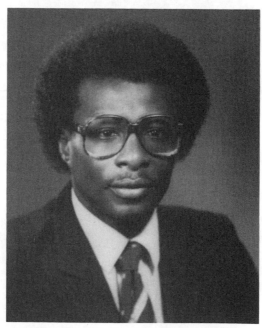

Cornell McBride Sr. with Afro in the 1970's

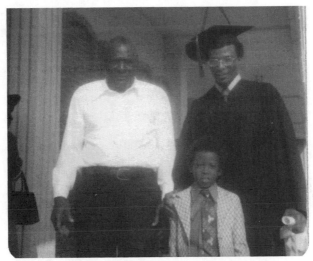

My father, Edward McBride and son, Cornell McBride Jr. at my
graduation from Pharmacy School

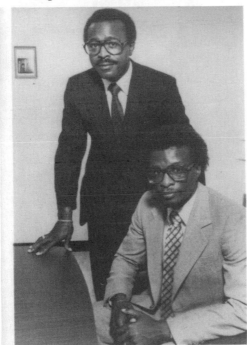

Cornell and Therman sporting Afros in the 1980's

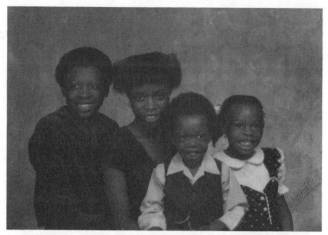

Early Family Portrait- Cornell Jr., Sheila, Andre, and Sholanda McBride

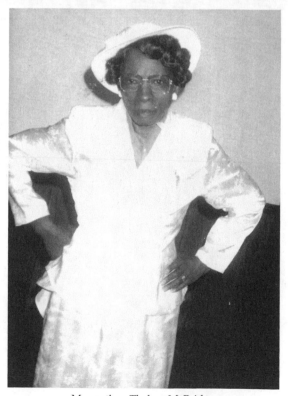

My mother, Thelma McBride

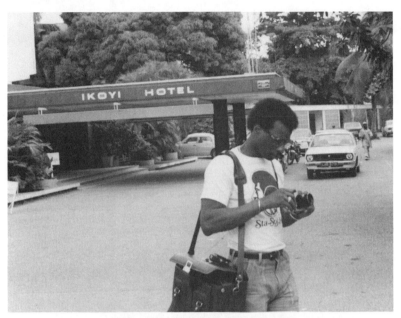

Cornell McBride Sr. in Nigeria 1979

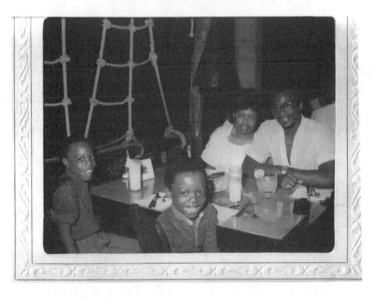

Sholanda, Andre, Harriet, and Cornell McBride Sr.
on vacation in Acapulco, Mexico

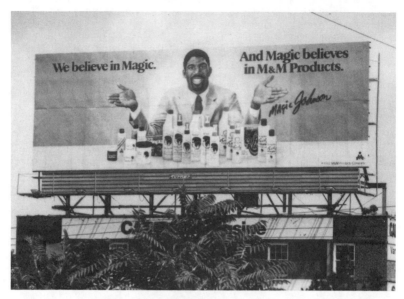

Billboard of Magic Johnson in London England

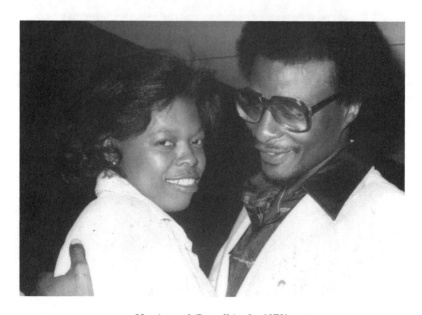

Harriet and Cornell in the 1970's

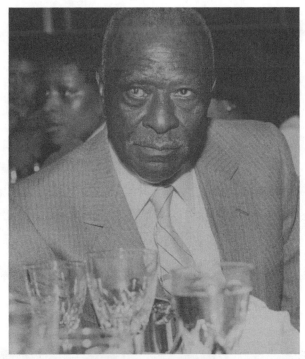

My father, Edward McBride

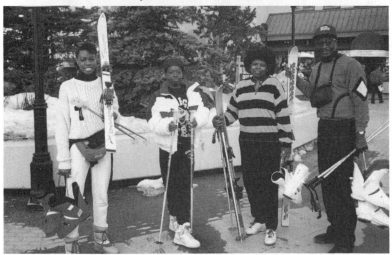

(L. TO R.) Sholanda McBride, Andre McBride, Harriet McBride, and
Cornell McBride Sr. on a ski trip

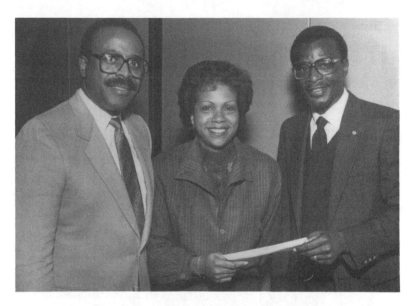

M & M Products makes a $10,000 contribution for famine relief in Ethiopia.
(L. TO R.) Therman McKenzie, Geraldine Thompson, and Cornell McBride Sr.

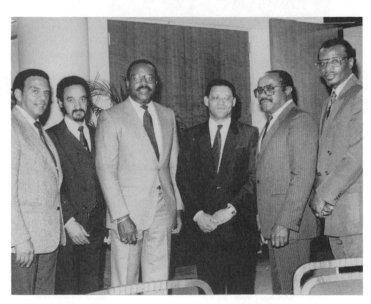

(L. TO R.) Andrew Young, Unknown Gentleman, Therman McKenzie, South
African Businessman, Carl Ware of Coca Cola, and Cornell McBride Sr.

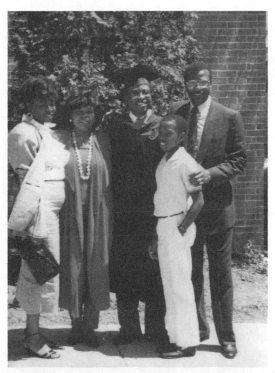

Sheila McBride, Harriet McBride, Cornell McBride Jr., (Graduating From Howard University), Andre McBride and Cornell McBride Sr.

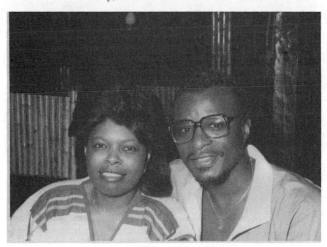

Harriet and Cornell in the 1980's

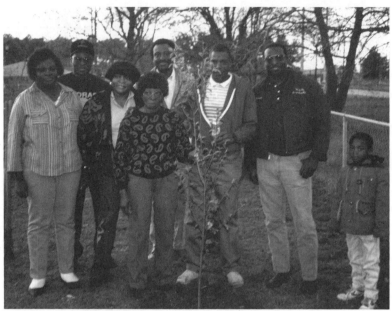

(L. To R.) Sister- Bernice, Myself, Sister- Rose, Mother- Thelma,
Brother- Eddie, Brother-Earl, Brother-Garfield

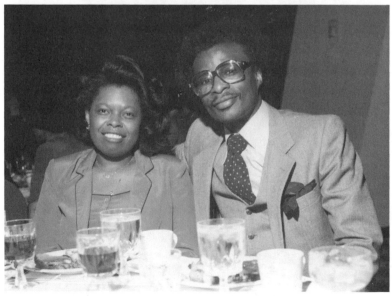

Harriet and Cornell McBride celebrating M & M Product's 10th Anniversary

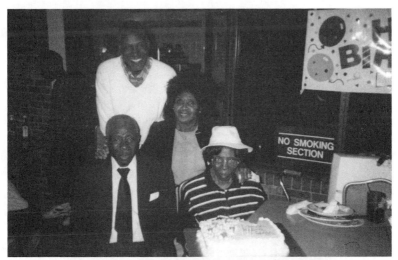

Uncle Freeman Jones (L.) Brother Earl (Standing), Aunt Ruby
and my mother, Thelma

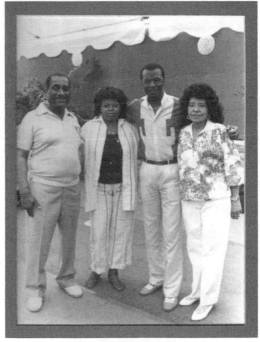

(L.TO R.) John Johnson of Ebony Magazine, Harriet McBride,
Cornell McBride Sr., and Mrs. Johnson

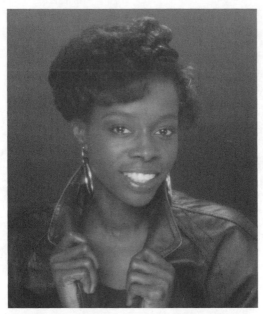

My deceased daughter, Sheila McBride

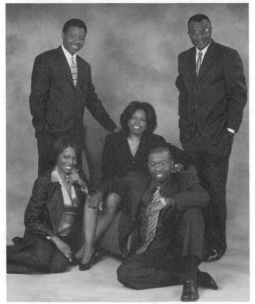

The McBride Family- (L. TO R.) Sholanda, Cornell Jr., Harriet, Andre, and Cornell Sr. (Photo by Ernest Washington at www.edupphoto.com)

Chapter 13: Taking Sta Sof Fro on the Road

"What if we leave Revco to work on M&M full time?" I asked Therman shortly after moving into my first home. "We could really build the brand, build the company. Now is the time to devote ourselves to the business full time." It was true. Though we had increased output at the new facility in order to meet demand, Therman and I were still technically working part time on new business and distribution since our daytime hours were spent as pharmacists at Revco. There had been pressure to go into M&M full time since Roosevelt left, because even with Roscoe, only part of our distribution was covered. There were still not enough products getting out the door to meet demand. My little home assembly line was wonderful, but we were stretched too thin.

"We could do that. It'd be a risk, but we could do it."

"We'll get a business loan, and expand—this time to a small plant. We'll start advertising."

Therman agreed, and so we went back to C&S

Bank, the regional Georgia-based institution where
Therman had secured his initial loan for M&M.

"Not yet. You need more business experience," the
loan officer told us. "You're off to a great start, there's
no doubt about that. But you should take some business classes. Try Southeastern Institute. They have
night classes. Just don't quit your day jobs yet."

The prospect of going back to school was not entic-
ing, and we were a little let down after feeling so excited about breaking out on our own. Worse yet, I practically cringed at the thought of adding yet another job
to my list. A job is what a business class would be, really. At the same time, however, I was excited by the idea
of learning more about building our business. Besides,
if that was what would get us a loan, then that's what
we would do.

Within a few months, we were back at the bank,
tired, but enriched by the experience. "Say, weren't
you the young men in here some months ago?" the
loan officer asked us as he came out to the bank's
lobby area to greet us.

"Yes, Sir. That was us," I answered. "You suggested business courses, and we took them. Now we're
back." I handed him our sales figures and projected
growth numbers for the coming year.

"We need to expand," I explained. "Again."

"Yes," Therman backed me up. "This business is
taking off day by day. We are bursting at the seams,
and if we can't get into a facility that can help us output to meet demand, we'll lose our customer base for
sure. We're doing really well, but we need some help
to get to the next level."

"We're ready to go into it full time," I offered. "We're ready to build this business."

"Let's talk," the loan officer said, and ushered us to his desk, where he offered us seats before sitting down himself. Then he pored over the paperwork I had given him. "It's promising. These numbers are very promising. There's no doubt about that. But there is still risk. You're unproven businessmen with no collateral."

"We're only looking for $5,000," Therman protested, emphasizing "only." It was a large amount of money for us, but we were positive M&M was good for it.

The loan officer frowned.

Therman did not give him any more time to think. "You took a chance on us once before. It paid off. Why not do it again?"

Still frowning, the loan officer looked up at Therman and me, as if seeing us for the first time. "I did? I thought I just gave you some advice."

Therman shook his head. "Before that. I came in. I was on my own, but looking for a small loan so I could contribute my half to starting up M&M Products. You authorized $500. I put $250 into M&M, and the other $250 into savings—just in case."

"Hold on. If I talked to you before, I've got your folder here somewhere." He shuffled papers on his desk, and then leaned over to look through a file drawer below. "McKenzie, right? Therman?" his muffled voice asked.

"That's right," Therman responded.

Finally, he found what he was looking for. "Here

we go," he said, reappearing in front of us. Then he glanced through a folder, and looked up at Therman. "Yup, it's right here. $500. And you paid it back within a month!"

"That's right," Therman concurred.

"And look here," the officer said, pointing at the folder. "You're a Mercer man!"

"Right again. We both are," Therman gestured at me. "Class of '73."

"So you are," he smiled. Abruptly, he stood up and put out his hand. "Congratulations, gentlemen."

Momentarily startled, we rushed to shake his hand. With that, we had ourselves a $5,000 signature loan based solely on our Mercer connection.

"One piece of advice, if I may."

We nodded, grateful for any words that would help us become as successful as possible.

"You both work as pharmacists, right?"

We nodded.

"And you want to leave to put everything into your company?"

We nodded again.

"One of you should stay at the pharmacy, and one should go full time into M&M."

"What?" Therman and I asked in unison. We had worked it all out. Both of us were leaving Revco.

"This is our business together," I protested.

The loan officer held up his hands to quiet us. "It is. I know. I am not suggesting you break apart the business, but you should be sensible. If you both leave your jobs, and M&M fails, you're both out of work. It's safer if one of you keeps his day job."

We agreed, finally, but the question was now, who's going to go with M&M whole hog?

On the drive back to my house, we discussed it. "You've got a family to consider," Therman offered.

"Yeah, and I appreciate that. But I've got more business experience than you do." It was true. Not only that, but I was older, more mature. Therman was the most self-assured guy I had ever met, and he was wonderful with people, always popular. He was also wiser and worldlier than his years, though he had never traveled beyond Georgia except to see his sister in Ohio once. So, it was not that Therman could not run the business—he was, after all, already running it jointly with me. But somehow, it just seemed like a risk I should be taking. After all, I had doggedly pursued starting the business to begin with, and so if it was going to fail, I wanted that failure to rest on my shoulders, not his.

We decided that Therman would stay at Revco until M&M was secure enough for both of us to leave. As it turned out, that security would be just around the corner. But when I told Harriet what I was doing, I did not know that. It was not easy breaking the news to my wife. This was one of only a few decisions I have made without consulting her first. Then when I did, I also picked a bad time.

I was bringing boxes into the basement from the car. Since I had quite a few, I cut a path through the lawn. Harriet came out to the porch when she heard me. "Cornell," she exclaimed. "I just finished re-seeding the lawn, and now you're walking back and forth all over it."

"Do you see those boxes on the curb? I still have those to carry in, and I already carried in half a dozen. Let me be."

The look in her eyes drilled two holes right through me. She was done talking about it and went back in side.

"You *what*?" she asked in disbelief when I told her later that evening after finishing up in the basement. "What do you mean you're leaving the pharmacy?"

"It's the only thing that makes sense."

Silence.

"Harriet, if I do not do this now, I might never do it. I might get stuck behind that counter, get complacent and then be afraid to leave. Besides, I do not have *time* to wait. I'm 30 years old already! I don't have time to waste."

Still angry, she said, "You think that this product is going to make you rich."

"Yup. Yes I do. But," I added with resolve, "we are not going to get rich with me behind the counter at Revco. I promise you that."

After some silence, she said, "As long as you take care of us, we're okay." And that was that.

The next day, I turned in my resignation. I was feeling light as air, looking forward with great anticipation to putting all my energies toward M&M. Word about my impending departure soon spread among my Revco colleagues and patients. Most were excited for me, but a few expressed reservations. I recall an older gentleman, a patient in his 70s, who waited for me to fill some prescriptions before taking me aside. "Son, tell me," he started, with deep concern in his voice.

"You say that you are going to give up your good job to work in your basement to sell hair products?" He sounded utterly incredulous.

"Yes, sir. That is what I intend to do."

"I wouldn't do that, if I were you, son," he continued, shaking his head. "You have a good job. A *good* job."

I thanked him for his concern, and told him I was not going to fail. I did not want to be disrespectful by arguing with him. After all, it occurred to me that, for his generation, a black man was lucky to have a job. He was a man born at the turn of the 20th century, barely 30 years after slavery ended. Careers, ownership, the sort of participation that white men historically took for granted just did not seem to be an option for the older generation of black men—even my generation was not entirely comfortable with creating their own opportunities, or seizing those that happened to come along. Many did not recognize them at all.

The prospect of ownership was just too alluring for me to pass by. Once I had conceived it, imagined that I could own my own company, it was something I had to make real for myself. As the elderly gentleman turned to leave, I called out to him. "If it doesn't work out, I can always come back." He smiled wistfully, and wished me well.

I left Revco in May of 1974. Early in the morning my first day with M&M Products, I set about planning our expansion outside of Atlanta. When we first started the business, we rented a post office box. I went to go check our mail. There were letters from all over Georgia, South Carolina, Florida, Alabama, North Carolina, and even up north, from places like Chicago and New York. They were all asking where they could find Sta Sof Fro in their cities and towns: "I have never found anything like this!" "My cousin brought some back from his trip to Atlanta. Now I want Sta Sof Fro." "I do not make a habit of writing letters to companies extolling the virtues of their products. But I have to say that I have never used a product before like Sta Sof Fro. Please inform me as to locations in my area where I may purchase more of this wonderful hair balm." "This product has made my hair so manageable, I can do so much more with it than I ever could." It was true, and as we would soon learn, Sta Sof Fro would revolutionize hair fashion by giving individuals and stylists more design freedom.

Letters like these had begun trickling in a few weeks earlier, and Therman and I discussed what to do. "Aren't we ready to go regional?" I asked, holding up a couple of letters. Sta Sof Fro is already making the rounds."

Therman agreed. "We're already all over Atlanta."

Now that I was completely immersed in M&M, it seemed logical to take the next step to do the work to put Sta Sof Fro in stores in the Southeast region. In the meantime, however, we had all these fan letters. Therman hit upon a terrific idea.

"We should answer them," he said. "But also go one better."

"How do you mean?" I asked, not excited about taking the time to write back to each person. Even though I knew what it must have taken to get them to write in the first place, those letters were starting to pile up. Besides, it was the face-to-face contact I enjoyed, not letter-writing.

"Let's go get some stationery made up with M&M letterhead," Therman continued. "Then we'll write an official letter thanking them for their correspondence, and pack some free bottles of Sta Sof Fro."

It was a brilliant idea. Until we could get the product to stores in their area, we would do by mail what we'd done on the streets of Atlanta: sample. They'd have some and maybe share some with their friends. Then, once we got into area salons, barbershops, beauty supply stores and drug stores, we could write them again and tell them where to find it.

It seemed that, almost as soon as I went into M&M full time, sales outgrew the McBride basement. It was time to make a choice: remain where we were and stop growing, or make the commitment to move to a professional facility where we could manufacture large quantities of inventory, have our offices, hire office and plant assistance, and ramp up a marketing strategy to increase distribution.

"Therman!" I marched up to the pharmacy counter at Revco where he was filling prescriptions. "Take off that coat, man, and come with me. We have business to attend to."

After fulfilling his two-week notice commitment, Therman left Revco in August of 1974, just a few months after I had left. Now, McKenzie and McBride were both full-time co-owners of M&M Products. We were ready to start looking for professional office and manufacturing space. In the meantime, however, there was still current demand to be met and more business to create.

Once we started brainstorming about responding

to the letter-writers, other ideas started streaming out. I snapped my fingers. "The military! Why didn't I think of that before? It's perfect!"

"The military?"

"Yes, of course. Think of all the bases in the Southeast alone." I started ticking off a few. "Fort Stewart in Savannah. Fort Jackson in Columbia, South Carolina. Fort McClellan in Alabama. Fort Gordon in Augusta. Andrews Air Force Base in D.C."

"Okay." Therman waited for me to explain.

"Post exchanges. They've all got 'em."

"What's a post exchange?"

"It's like a general store. Think about it. A military base is like a small city, pretty much self-contained. So, they're going to have places where folks buy necessities. Imagine, if we can get Sta Sof Fro in a few of these places, I bet it'll get hot real quick."

Therman liked the idea. He also liked the angle of using my status as a veteran to get us a foot in the door. "One question. Who the heck do you call?"

It was a fair question. We think of the military as being separate from any part of civilian life—so separate that we forget they have to supply their personnel with many of the same products civilians use everyday.

Somehow I got a hold of a catalog that had information on how the military contracts with vendors to supply post exchanges. I found out the buying center was in Alabama, and contacted the man in charge. We set up an appointment, readied our presentation and then headed down to see him.

Once we sat down in his office, he began peppering

us with questions. "So, how long has M&M been in business?"

Concerned he would shy away from our relative inexperience, we decided to steer the conversation toward what was really important: what a great product we had. "If I may," I started, "let me first tell you a bit about our product. That's where the really interesting conversation is to be had."

Soon enough, we had him engrossed in just how popular Sta Sof Fro had become. "It's revolutionary, really," Therman said enthusiastically.

I held up a handful of letters we'd received. "These are just what we got yesterday. Ten letters. That means that there are ten times that many people who didn't write, but still want our product."

"Especially black men," Therman interjected. "They haven't had a product before now that let them comb their hair while keeping it soft."

The buyer smiled and ran his hand over his buzz cut. "Well, I don't quite have that problem."

"I didn't used to, either," I said. "I was an airman until '67."

"You were an enlisted man?" he asked, his eyes lighting up. "Well, heck, it's a pleasure to meet a fellow veteran." He stood up and reached out to shake my hand.

"Likewise."

"And now you're a pharmacist."

"We both are, Therman and I. And, we developed Sta Sof Fro for our own hair. As you can see, it's worked wonders on mine, and I've only been using it for about two years."

"It is a nice head of hair," he agreed. "Afro is what you call it, right?"

"That's right," I smiled. "And when I left the service, my hair was dry and hard like you wouldn't believe. I had trouble growing it, too."

"So, you think there's a market here? But none of the men have those Afro hairstyles."

"Short hair, long hair. Doesn't matter. It does what it says, makes your hair soft. A man with any hair height appreciates that," I responded. "I've got a few letters from military men here, too. Some came across it while in Atlanta. Others got it from friends. Believe me, there's a demand here, for sure."

"Tell you what," the buyer offered. "Let's try you on ten bases across the Southeast."

Therman and I looked at each other, and nodded.

There were separate purchase orders for each base. The procedure was that the buyer filled out the order, and then the vendor shipped the product to each post exchange. Then the buyer would track sales and decide whether or not to order more, less, or take the product off the shelves.

We took our purchase orders and headed back to Atlanta. But rather than simply shipping boxes to each base, we followed everyone up with a personal visit. Flashing the purchase order at the guard gate, we gained access to the various bases. I almost fell out of the car laughing the first time a guard waved us through. Therman thought he was saluting us, so he saluted back, and the guard did not quite know what to do.

Once on base, he made a beeline to a formation conducting drill practice, hands full of samples. As the company marched, shouting, "I don't know what I've been told!" Therman tried to hand out bottles. Fortunately, I was able to call him off before the drill sergeant caught a look. There was no doubt Therman was tenacious!

"Come on, man," I said, still recovering from the guard gate salute. "Let's get on to the exchange. We can set up there." And that's how we started spreading Sta Sof Fro across the Southeast. We knew that from there, military folks would spread the word far and wide.

And then, there we were, near the end of 1974. Barely two years had passed since I first started handing out samples of an unnamed hair softener while students at Mercer University. Not even six months had elapsed since I left Revco to work on M&M full time. Now we were ready to establish a company headquarters for M&M Products in buildings that weren't basements of apartments and houses. If nothing else told us, the numbers did.

One night, toward the end of 1974, Therman and I sat in my kitchen at the breakfast table and crunched the numbers.

"That can't be right," Therman said in disbelief. "Check that out."

I looked at the paperwork. Then I smiled. "Mm-hmm. That's $100,000 in sales."

"If I did not see it with my own eyes, I would not believe it."

Doing the calculations had not convinced me that we'd reached so much success in so short a time. It was seeing the inventory, packing the boxes for distribution, and visiting the stores that told me how well we were doing. The paperwork only backed up what I already knew. And what I knew was $100,000 in sales for 1974.

Chapter 14: The Money Train Takes Off

Therman and I always said, "If we take care of the business, the business will take care of us." We were fastidious in our commitment to grow the company, not our personal fortunes. The company came first. When we left Revco, we paid ourselves a salary, but we kept it the same amount—$15,000 a year—we made as pharmacists. That was a decent amount of money in the mid-1970s, and we saw no reason to pay ourselves more until M&M was a solidly established company. Consequently, we did not enrich ourselves at the expense of the company. This was one of the key features of our remarkable and rapid success.

As a result of our fiscal discipline, every year after 1974 until the early 1980s, when we reached $45-$50 million, sales practically doubled. By 1979, less than six years after we first began handing out samples to get our product onto shelves, M&M Products reached about $18 million in sales. Our profits, inventory and production were turning over so fast that it was not long before we owned the market.

But there, sitting at that table at the end of 1974, it was easy to question the numbers. I might have done so myself if I had not seen the inventory, watched it in distribution and kept track of the monthly sales. I grasped the volume we sold by watching the boxes go out the door and visiting our customers. If I could see with my own eyes the totality of what we were doing, I could understand why the numbers were what they were.

Though it was not hard to see the volume of inventory we were putting out, it was increasingly hard to see the floor of my basement. The space became so cramped that we had to be careful where we moved an elbow when working on the assembly line. One false move, and a column of product-filled boxes could come crashing down.

"Watch it, man!" I cried out as Therman attempted to pass behind me one day in early 1975. "That whole wall is about to fall."

"I am watching it," Therman snapped back, "but I can barely see in front of me."

Though it was clear M&M Products Company had outgrown the basement of my house, we had been too busy finding new outlets for our product to figure out what to do about it. Besides, drawing up the plans and finding funding so that we could move into a full-fledged manufacturing plant and office suite was not my idea of a good time. But I knew that I had to adjust my thinking to accommodate the reality of the business. Had we remained in the basement of my house, the business would have stagnated.

"Come on," Therman put down his box. "We're going to find us a place."

I agreed. We sat down and discussed the next phase of M&M Products, which included expanding our operation and pouring money into advertising.

"If we stay idle," I said, "the competition will eventually find us. We've already gotten some attention, and we have to find a way to get way out ahead if we are going to keep from getting crushed."

"As soon as legislation passes on listing the ingredients," Therman agreed, "and we know it's going to, there's going to be a whole wave on top of us."

He was right. When we put out our first bottles of Sta Sof Fro, we were not required to list the ingredients. We knew, however, because we followed the news closely, that it was only a matter of time before the government passed legislation requiring the contents be listed on all product containers, including hair-care items. When that happened, the competition would hustle to copy our formula. This meant we had to expand our market nationwide fast, which in turn meant a major increase in advertising and a strategy to make every advertising penny count.

Needless to say, there was a lot of pressure not just to keep up with demand, but also to expand our sales base so that we could dominate the market before our competitors got hold of our ingredients. Two main forces were driving our thinking as we looked toward 1975: first, the sheer volume of demand for the product, which had got us to the $100,000 sales point to begin with. Second, there was our race against time. Once a law passed requiring the listing of ingredients on packaging, the market would start flooding with

Sta Sof Fro knock-offs. We had to corner the soft hair market before that happened.

Another force that drove me on was my burning desire to become a success. Though I grew up not knowing what shape that would take, once I had developed the formula that became Sta Sof Fro, I knew I had found it. If I learned everything I needed to know about business and the hair-care industry, M&M Products would be the success I had dreamed of since I was a boy.

The following May, in 1975, we moved into a 3,000-square-foot building on Brown's Mill Road in Atlanta, signing a two-year lease on the property that included offices and a lab for developing new formulas and manufacturing Sta Sof Fro. Before long, we had to buy a trailer to store additional materials, and we parked it on site. Therman and I picked out side-by-side offices, and we hired the first of our office staff, longtime friend and fellow pharmacist, Annie Washington. She took on multiple roles that smoothed the transition from two-man operation to a carefully constructed company: executive assistant, office manager and administrator. "Well," I smiled to myself as I entered my new office for the first time. "I suppose I have myself an executive job."

I was 32 years old, and would be a millionaire in three years. Therman and I were in the zone, to use a sports analogy. We felt confident about the future, but we had no time to enjoy the moment. There was too much to do, and we were determined not to be simply riding the rocket that was taking off. We wanted to make sure it was pointed in the right direction, and so we knew we had to be organized in both our current business practices and our plans for the future of M&M. Part of that organization was determined by how successful Sta Sof Fro was, and Sta Sof Fro's success was due in large part to marketing and advertising. The advertising, in turn, was based on a strategy we developed early on in 1975.

Sampling had been a successful way of generating excitement about the product. We'd seen that firsthand throughout Atlanta, and then when we went regional by way of the military. Advertising was another way to create excitement, and Therman and I learned a great deal about how to advertise effectively. A mutual acquaintance put Therman and me in touch with a man named Bob Cheney, who had a small advertising agency and could help us develop more television commercials. We started working with him on advertising right away, knowing that this was the new version of sampling. Therman and I had been good marketers, but now we had the capital to be even better.

From the beginning, we put 15 %-20 % of our gross sales back into advertising. We began in 1975 with the local radio station in Atlanta, WAOK. In those days, there was only one black station, and, like all the music stations at the time, it was AM.

We set up a meeting with WAOK's advertising sales manager and went in prepared. We had our sales pitch down pat, and though we were there as clients, we still felt like we were selling our product. Because of that, we brought along samples and T-shirts, and then sat down to tell him our story. He was initially impressed, and then we handed him a bottle.

"Go ahead and try a little," I said, smiling. "You will not be disappointed."

Like most of the guys at that station, the sales manager had a substantial Afro. "Here," he said, passing us a folder. "These are the various packages we offer. You'll see we write the copy, which you approve, and then there are rates listed for the various broadcast times." Then he stood up. "Look through those, and I'll be right back." He held up the bottle of Sta Sof Fro and flashed a smile. "I've heard about this stuff."

He emerged a minute later with a big grin on his face, and brought me and Therman around the station to meet some of the other employees. "You've got to try this," he cooed, wafting his hands across the top of his Afro. "Smooth and soft!" Soon enough, most of the station's employees had tried Sta Sof Fro, and those who didn't were already frequent users of the product.

Before we left the station, the main DJ, "Jive Master," walked in. When he got hold of Sta Sof Fro, he did not stop talking about it. "Let's do some On-Air with this," he said.

Therman and I looked at each other. "Excuse us?" I asked.

"Get on the air and get people talking about this—" he looked at the bottle and continued, "this Sta Sof Fro, Man! Where did you get this?"

"We made it," I replied.

DJ JM looked at us and nodded. "Cool," he purred.

Through DJ Jive Master we learned about soliciting DJs at other stations to do live commercials, and he always gave us extra time, talking on and on about M&M's products.

The sales manager liked Sta Sof Fro so much that he threw in some advertising extras. The morning and afternoon drive times, especially just before the weekend, were the most valuable advertising slots. Most people did their shopping on the weekends, and typically had present of mind what they had heard on the radio. We were given additional air time at no extra cost, along with some valuable advertising education.

We learned not only about drive time and end-of-week advertising, we also learned about whom we should advertise to. Though Sta Sof Fro was developed primarily for men, we learned that women were generally the purchasers of the household. Consequently, we advertised to that demographic. In addition, we learned how to get advertising agency discounts that radio stations included in their packages for large companies, even though we did not have an advertising agency working for us.

After we got Sta Sof Fro on WAOK, we began branching out. First we went to WSOK in Savannah, and then to Birmingham, Alabama. Soon enough, we were broadcasting all over the Southeast. At the same time, we were still traveling from city to city, finding some stores interested in stocking our product, and others willing only to take it on consignment. Wherever we found resistance, we increased our advertising so that the next time we arrived at a store that had not wanted to stock Sta Sof Fro, they were more than pleased to see us. Some vendors did not even wait for us to return, but would call us asking to send the product.

We always kept moving. If Johnson Products'

salesmen called on 10 stores a day, we called on 30. They wore nice suits, but we wore charm, and in the end, our hunger for success was stronger than theirs. After all, we owned our own company, and the suits just had 9-to-5 jobs. Sure, they had a steady paycheck, but we were *owners*. By growing our company it was like we were growing ourselves, feeding off of each new sale like it was our life sustenance.

Advertising sales managers soon learned to love when we came calling. We spent more than the average company, usually 13 weeks of advertising, and had our spots in heavy rotation—somewhere in the neighborhood of 30 to 50 a week. We could see, toward the end of 1975, that we would exceed $800,000 in sales—almost ten times what we ended at the year before. Therman and I decided to spend a significant portion of our revenue on advertising—beyond our original percentage.

"I have been giving this some thought," I told him one day in the fall of 1975. We liked to saunter into each other's offices sometimes just to jaw a little. Although we spent a significant portion of our lives together in the past few years, we liked checking in when there were new ideas. We were each other's best sounding board. "Our plan is to corner the market."

"Right," Therman nodded.

"We are on our way to doing that. But we can do better."

"I'm listening."

"The accountant says we will have more taxes than we counted on. He just asked if we had any other expenses we could count in this quarter."

"I know it," Therman replied in frustration. "We sweat to make the money and the government just takes it away."

I shook my head. "No, man. We can make this work for us. Fourth quarter spending. If we spend the difference on advertising in November, we won't have those taxes due come spring."

Therman's face brightened. "I like it."

"And that's not all. The more we spend, the better hold we have on the market—"

"And," Therman finished the thought for me, "the easier it will be to keep out the competition."

We might not have had the financial clout of, say, Johnson Products, but we could outspend them on advertising. They had so many products to advertise, they could only allocate a certain amount for each market. M&M Products, on the other hand, had only one. I was developing a shampoo to go with Sta Sof Fro, but at the time, we could put $100,000 toward advertising for the year for our single product, while other companies could not. Then, when we saw big profits toward the end of the year, we could spend another $50,000.

"It's perfect," Therman beamed. "This also sets us up to come out big early next year." It was true. Advertising late in the year led to large sales figures in the first quarter of the New Year. Our January and February sales took off, and our previous tax year burden was lessened.

Therman, Cheney and I worked out how and when to advertise on television to get the most for our money. We knew we needed to target mothers, so we bought time during the soap operas. For the men, we focused on wrestling events, and for both men and women, we advertised on "Soul Train" and local dance shows patterned after it, and we advertised on Saturday morning cartoon shows. We bought on the local network affiliates, but we also found stations that reached a broader audience.

BET was just starting out then, and though most people thought cable television was pointless, its founder, Robert Johnson, was a visionary. At the time, their programming was not targeted, but since the network itself was for black audiences, and since they solicited our advertising, we spent some there. Ted Turner's Channel 17 was another advertising outlet. It showed only movies, but it reached all over the Southeast, and so we got a larger audience than the local advertising price we paid.

With Cheney's help, and that of director and photographer Dan Moore, who later went on to found the African American Museum Apex in Atlanta, we were able to shoot some successful ads. By the end of the decade, we began advertising in *Jet* and *Ebony* magazines, and received good responses from the billboard campaign we did with Cheney. It featured a toddler with a huge Afro photographed from a side view, bending over with his face toward the camera. Beneath him the sign read, "Sta Sof Fro makes hair as soft as a baby's..."

Cornell Jr. was about 9 years old at the time and very cute. He also had a fine, round Afro. We created a commercial around him, in which he sits on a stool holding up a bottle of Sta Sof Fro. "I used to hate to

comb my hair. But one day my mom gave me this bottle. Now I love to comb my hair." He did quite well
with his lines, too! Later, we created another ad with
Cornell Jr. and an actress playing his mom.

Watching other companies' advertising during that
period also taught us about their advertising strategies. George Johnson, the head of Johnson Products,
was considered the godfather of the industry. Johnson
Products was the premier black hair-care company at
that time and was the first black company to do many
things. It was the first to be traded on the American
Stock Exchange. It also was an early sponsor of "Soul
Train," and often on the cutting edge of advertising in
the market George Johnson helped create. It was
George who started mass distribution of black products, including retailing a home kit for permanent hair
straightening. He created a commercial for Afro Sheen,
using African dialect, which I believe was one of the
very first to do so. Like the commercials they pio-
neered, Johnson Products were also always tastefully
packaged. They took the industry to another level, out
of mom and pop stores, and brought lots of visibility
to the industry. I was proud to become friends with
George, who is now retired, and grateful for what I
learned from his groundbreaking work.

There was so much that Therman and I figured out
as we went along. We got good advice here and there,
and we always capitalized on it with our own instincts
and creativity. We always worked together as a team,
playing off each other's strengths, knowing when to
let the other take the lead in negotiations, or when to
provide back-up because we knew that the two of us

together were greater than one of us alone. Those five years went faster than a bullet train, but they were exciting and remarkably rewarding because of the effort we put into it.

I read everything I could get my hands on concerning business management, advertising and entrepreneurship. I wanted to understand every aspect of business. There is no end to learning, and part of that process means asking questions, accepting criticism and being open to change. I never wanted to reach a point of complacency. The ideas I read about helped me crystallize ways of behaving that I had grown up with, and also showed me how personal and character-based business is. Business is not just about making a buck, it's about doing right and good, having a company of character. This stood me in good stead when I worked on developing new products, and although many people do not give the ethics of hair care much thought, I was sensitive to the political, social and cultural significance of black hair.

It might seem strange to people to think about hair in political terms, but just as women wearing "bloomers" in the 19th century was an important social, cultural and political statement, black hairstyles also heralded or manifested important ideas. When West Africans and blacks from other lands were forcibly removed from their native lands, they were stripped of everything. Even seemingly unimportant implements such as combs were left behind, and photos reveal men and women with bald patches and unkempt hair. Part of our human dignity is bound up with details of our lives, such as being able to wash ourselves and brush our hair. Ever since then, what black people did with their hair was significant.

I wanted to make sure I respected that significance attached to hair, and so every product M&M put out had to meet the highest standards. At the end of the '70s, while developing a product for the curl market, I saw it caused too much breakage. I shut down development, but another company picked it up and made a lot of money—in the short run. Thankfully, that company later went out of business.

As part of my efforts at self-improvement, I also sought out business seminars and workshops through the American Management Association (AMA). Such workshops and seminars proved so helpful that I would eventually travel across the country to Stanford University to attend. I also became involved in the black chamber of commerce, the NAACP and other organizations, and though Therman was not initially interested in community and political involvement, he did support the philanthropic endeavors I got M&M Products into. In fact, Therman became known as the one at M&M with the deep pockets. "Giving back to the community that gave so much to us," was our company's charity motto, and we incorporated our community involvement into our advertising. The tag at the end of our commercials was, "From the people who know your hair, and care." And we meant it. We did not want simply to be a company that happened to be based in Atlanta; we wanted to be a company that made a difference in the community in which we lived, and in which we had a stake as citizens. We would tag the end of commercials with a five second public service announcement, such as, "Don't forget to get out and vote this November."

Not long after, I joined several up-and-coming black businessmen, including Nate Goldstein, Mac Wilburn, Joe Hudson and Preston Torrance and started a businessmen's activist group so that our voices could be heard in the community. We eventually became instrumental in helping to elect Maynard Jackson to office as Atlanta's mayor. Before we knew it, we were helping out Andy Young, and making significant financial contributions to political campaigns. Today, Nate runs Atlanta-based Gourmet Services, a food services company with major college and university accounts across the country. Mac owns a number of businesses in the Atlanta airport, and Joe, who worked at one time for Gourmet Services, is a consultant in Atlanta. Preston was a professor at Atlanta University, and he hosted most of our meetings, along with various events and parties for Atlanta luminaries. From the beginning of M&M's meteoric rise those were heady days. All the while, we kept building our company.

Chapter 15: Structuring the Dream

While we were working out of the Browns Mill Road building, Therman and I had worn all the hats: research and development, marketing and advertising, sales and finance. Thankfully, Annie Washington kept the offices running smoothly. We also were fortunate to connect with a number of talented people who helped us grow M&M, but by and large, it was a two-man operation. With the rapid expansion we experienced due to the popularity of Sta Sof Fro, however, we knew the company would soon need a formal structuring, which meant the creation of departments and the people to staff them. But before that could happen, we had to find bigger office, warehouse and manufacturing space once again.

"It's time," Therman smiled, leaning back in his chair. "Again." We were sitting in his office in 1976, planning for the coming year. From the initial $500 loan we got to start M&M Products, we generated about $30,000 in sales, while still working as pharmacists in 1973. The $5,000 signature loan we got from the same bank was parlayed into $300,000 by the end of 1974. In 1976, we realized that we had outgrown our 3,000-square- foot office and manufacturing space, and that once again, it was time to move up to the next level. Our sales were $300,000 in 1975, and $800,000 in 1976.

I was on top of the world. Harriet, Sheila, Cornell Jr., and Sholanda welcomed André to the family that year. Harriet and I were enjoying the fruits of our labors. We had four beautiful and talented children, a solid relationship, a nice new home, and a sense of security that came as a reward for all our efforts.

Harriet and I had sold our first house, and moved farther out to the suburbs of DeKalb County, into a lovely five-bedroom ranch-style house. The previously all-white subdivisions were increasingly integrated, and we were the third black family to move into our neighborhood. I remember the day we drove up to the house for the first time. I felt such pride at being able to move into a larger house, to have some property and give each of our kids their own bedroom.

As it turned out, not all of our neighbors were that excited. The first time I went out to my yard to mow my lawn, I saw one of my new neighbors, an older white man, working along the fence line. So, I rode my tractor mower over and waved hello. The man did not flinch, but I knew he had seen me. In all the time we were neighbors, he never said "hi," and never said "bye," and never once acknowledged any of us. As I rode away, I thought, "I don't know how you're doing, but I'm doing extremely well. You might not like the color of my skin, but I have two brand-new cars in the garage, and a brand-new boat parked in the driveway." Eventually, the man moved away. Our community, South DeKalb County, Georgia, became the county with the second highest per capita income area among African Americans in the entire country, and we were happy living there.

With my family settled into our new home, I began thinking about the house that I had promised my mother about 20 years ago. I called my parents with the good news of our business success.

"Mom," I said. "How big do you want your house?"

"What are you talking about?" I heard her soft voice on the other end of the line. "What house?"

"Do you remember a promise I made to you when I was 10?"

There was silence as she paused to recollect. Then she responded, a smile in her voice. "Yes, yes I do, now that you mention it. Is that what you mean?"

"That's right."

"Cornell," she said breathlessly, with a mixture of surprise and pride. "You were just a boy. I had forgotten about that, and I would have thought you did, too."

"No," I answered softly. "I have not forgotten about that promise even for one day."

"Cornell, you don't need to build me a house for me to be proud of you. I have always been proud of you."

"Mom, I have not forgotten. Well, I'm still planning on building you that house someday." That dream would come true in 1981.

In addition to the growth in my personal life, M&M

was also on solid ground after only three years in business. We had our advertising in place. The shampoo I had developed the previous year was out now and doing well, and recently we brought out Sta Sof Fro Intensive Conditioner. That, too, was performing solidly. I had modeled the shampoo on Revlon's Milk Plus 6, which had flopped miserably on the general market, but did very well in the ethnic market. They decided to bring it out exclusively for the ethnic market and renamed it Cream of Nature. At a Society of Cosmetic Chemists meeting, I had met the chemist who created Revlon's product, who told me the compound he used, JR-400, was a detangling conditioner. I decided to reformulate the product, using JR-400 as a main ingredient. The result was our version, Sta Sof Fro Shampoo, and it did very well in the black hair-care market.

With that success, I was eager to get into development more intensely, and work on both more companion products for Sta Sof Fro and entirely new lines. Doing so would require more space than the 3,000 square feet we had at Browns Mill Road. So, when Therman told us it was time to move, I was all for it. "You're right," I agreed. "It's not just the current inventory we've got. If we're going to develop more products, we need more lab and production space."

Therman and I turned to Trust Company Bank. It was there we first met Paul Turner, who would soon join us as Director of Finance at our new location. With his help we obtained a $50,000 SBA loan that allowed us to move into larger facilities and buy new equipment.

Once at the Royal Drive location, Therman and I had to ramp up structuring both the corporate and manufacturing sides of M&M Products. Annie Washington moved with us to continue as office manager. We brought over Paul Turner, the man from Trust Company Bank who arranged the $50,000 loan for us to move. It would be his job to make sure we did not overspend, and it would prove to be a difficult task. Therman and I were eager to grow the company to $100 million, and were ready to spend in order to get there. Paul, a slender, soft-spoken man, was persuasive and continually offered good financial advice.

"Eli is willing to come over," Therman told me in late 1978.

"That's good news!" Eli McKenzie, Therman's brother, had a Ph.D. in chemistry. Not only were we lucky to recruit him, but I was happy to have family and friends from the community working with us. Eli was willing to quit his job to come over to M&M, and we were grateful.

"He doesn't know about manufacturing," Therman continued, "but he'll learn fast." Therman was right. Eli proved to be a terrific director of manufacturing, and did a lot to help build the company by organizing our manufacturing division. He was fastidious about formula precision, and worked to create a number of products for the curl maintenance line we developed and put out under the Sta Sof Fro, and later, Soft 'n Free brands.

We also landed Joyce McGriff as our director of market research, whom we managed to hire away from the giant Coca-Cola company; Mack Hunter as our corporate attorney; and Mitch McKinney to direct sales. Mack was a few years ahead of us at Fort Valley

State College, and also from Therman's hometown. Mitch came over from a competitor, and had lots of contacts in the marketplace. He opened new doors to get our products into stores that previously did not carry our brand, and he found terrific sales people. Along with Darlene Hall, who was our first advertising and marketing manager, Mitch was important in impacting sales. Darlene advanced the marketing department—doing a terrific job of implementing our ideas and generating new ones. But we knew that marketing was crucial to M&M's future, and so required experience that Darlene did not have. We hired Ed Rutland as marketing manager to work with Darlene Hall. Although Darlene had been indispensable to positioning M&M's products, Ed had an M.B.A. and more extensive experience, and so we put him at the head of the department. Darlene took exception to this decision, and let Therman and I know.

"I have seniority," she insisted, when we brought her into my office and told her of Ed's hiring.

"Darlene, I know. No one knows more than Therman and me what you've done for this company."

"It doesn't look like it to me," she said indignantly.

"Look," Therman said. "Even considering what you've accomplished, you don't have enough experience yet to take things to the next level. Work with Ed, learn what it takes, and then you're next in line." Therman and I wholeheartedly believed in our employees, and supported them in their work. But at the level of corporate structuring, we had to look outside until our current employees developed the skills and experience to take over executive positions.

She grudgingly accepted our decision, but the relationship between her and Ed was not a happy one, and not without good reason. Ed had some good ideas, but they did not come through. Sometimes that failure was on Ed, and sometimes not. He worked, for example, to secure Michael Jackson as a spokesperson for M&M Products. We set up a meeting with Jackson's people in Los Angeles, but when Ed flew out there, they were upset that Therman and I had not taken the meeting ourselves. Then they said Jackson would promote our products if we put his photo on the product. "No way," Therman and I said when Ed called with the Jackson camp's proposal. "We're not going to compromise M&M's brand independence." So, that was the end of that. Ed came home, and we moved on. Later, when Jackson's head got burned in a frightening accident that happened while shooting a Pepsi commercial, we were quietly relieved he was not using Sta Sof Fro.

Other marketing ventures under Ed's direction did not work out, and eventually, he was released from M&M. All the while, demand for M&M products grew by leaps and bounds.

We knew all along that, although we had to increase manufacturing to keep up with demand, we had to make sure that demand kept rising, and that meant extensive marketing. Advertising had been fueled by the initial success of Sta Sof Fro, and then the advertising itself fueled our expansion. It was not long before manufacturing shifts at the plant increased from one shift to three. We barely had a moment to let the machines cool down every day.

The new facility on Royal Drive in Atlanta was
10,000 square feet, with additional space next door, if
needed. It did not take long before we were occupying
30,000 square feet. We made our landlord very, very
happy. Eventually, we had 27,000 more square footage
than we had over on Browns Mill Road, so that we had
multiple warehouses for supplies and inventory. No
longer could I walk into a single room and see what was
what. Though I had learned quickly about computer
tracking of sales and inventory after we moved into the
Browns Mill Road offices, I still felt most confident
when I could see the inventory with my own eyes, I
could see how sales were going. With things so spread
out at Royal Drive, I felt uneasy for the first time, as if I
was losing control of what Therman and I had created.
How could I keep track of what we were making and
what was going out the door and onto store shelves?

I wandered down to the warehouses when we first
settled into Royal Drive, and tried to take it all in. I
stood in front of the enormous buildings and realized
at that moment that there was more inventory and
more supplies than I could see with just one look. I
knew that people were busy in their offices doing
work that Therman and I had done virtually alone. I
felt out of touch, distanced from the details. Now, people would report to me, offer their expert advice, and
expect me to sign off on it. But how could I do that
when I would not know what was going on?

I moped around for the rest of that day. At dinner
that night, Harriet asked if I was feeling all right.
"Yeah," I said. "Just a little tired."

The next morning, my waking thought was, "Pull

it together, man! You have got to rise to this challenge. It's sink or swim." I practically ran to my office that morning, determined to learn in a new way. With managers running various departments, there was now a step between the guy on the line and me. I had to learn how the managers ran their departments, how the staff understood their jobs, and in turn, make sure that the higher-ups knew how the smallest details of the process worked.

With so much to do, and with my resolve to adapt to this new environment, my worry soon faded. And, if I thought that the past few years had gone by quickly, everything that happened from the moment we moved to Royal Drive, through the early 1980s was, in comparison, a blur. It was a period of constant change and adjustment, and I knew I had better be ready for the challenge.

As we filled out departments at M&M Products, I decided to lend a hand wherever I was most needed. When manufacturing had trouble keeping up with demand, and we knew we needed more equipment to increase production, I took Colonel Duke Nelson, my next-door neighbor who became an assistant to Dr. Eli McKenzie, around the country to various auctions to buy equipment. Colonel Nelson was United States Army all the way. Though already retired when I met him, Colonel Nelson exuded strict discipline, and that carried over to our offices. Once the equipment purchases were accomplished, and that department was on track, I turned my attention elsewhere, and so on down the line. Between the two of us, Therman and I covered every facet of M&M's planning, development,

production and sales. We decided to divide up reporting responsibilities. I covered marketing, research and
development and manufacturing, while Therman
guided finance, human resources and legal.

In addition to building our corporate structure, we
established M&M Products internationally. In 1979, we
began selling in Europe, the Caribbean and Africa. In
Europe, a couple of American basketball players from
Georgia were selling Sta Sof Fro, and Therman and I
took our first-ever European trip to meet with them. A
London firm, Dyke and Dryden, eventually became
M&M's UK distributor.

From Europe we flew on to Africa. A Nigerian businessman, who came across Sta Sof Fro and who, like
everyone else who tried it, thought it was revolutionary.
"I want to build a manufacturing facility," he told us in
clipped English when we first spoke with him over the
phone. "Come, and I will show you what I want to do."

Going to Africa was eye opening in a number of
ways. I expected to be greeted with open arms,
throngs of Africans just waiting to meet me. Instead,
people were struggling just to survive, and I was just
another person in the crowd. When we arrived at customs in Nigeria with our samples, a large, severe-look-
ing customs official in a military uniform barked at
Therman and me. "What's in the box?"

We looked up at him meekly. "Samples," we
squeaked meekly.

"Open the box!" he boomed. Several other officials
came over, and they tore open our samples box.

Once they were through, the officer's booming
voice came at us again, his accent sharp. "You pay
some munn-ee! *Munn-ee!*"

"What?" I asked. I soon learned that many people were looking for a "dash," and they were very up front about demanding it. Therman and I paid our unofficial customs tax, which the large man easily pocketed.

As part of my assimilation to Nigerian business practices, I had to get used to "go slows." Therman and I had a meeting with our new business contact, and we waited patiently in the hotel's foyer promptly at 9 a.m., when we were to be picked up by Mundi, our driver. An hour and a-half later, no Mundi. I was really angry, having strained my eyes looking at each approaching car to see if it was ours, and slowly sweating through my nice three-piece suit. "Where is this guy?" I growled at Therman.

"I don't know. Let me call the office." Therman went off to call our contact's office, and came back shortly. "It must be a 'go slow,'" he said matter-of-factly.

"A what?"

"A 'go slow.' It's a traffic jam."

Apparently, the traffic lights often went out in those days, and cars just bottlenecked on the already heavily trodden roads.

Finally, Mundi showed up at 11. He got out of his car and moved to take our briefcases. "Mundi," I said jabbing my finger at my wristwatch. "Do you know what time it is?"

Without missing a beat, Mundi said, "Ha, ha, ha, Master Sir, but this is not America." He kept moving around the car and got in. Therman and I quickly followed. I had learned my lesson. In the end, our Africa trip was both successful and deeply meaningful to me.

Our Blow Out Relaxer, used primarily by men, was a hit on our trip to Nigeria—it was doing well back in the States, but I don't think anyone in Africa had ever experienced anything like it. When we first got there, we were put in a hotel we did not like. There was a nice Holiday Inn, but it was booked solid. So, armed with Sta Sof Fro T-shirts and products, we bribed the guys at the front desk to get us rooms. "Do you want to change your hair?" we asked.

"What? Why?" they answered, perplexed.

"We can make it big," we said, miming a large Afro. "It will make your hair stand out."

In the end, they decided to go for it, and they were thrilled. Half-inch Afros became full three inches! "A miracle!" they cried. Before we knew it, guys were beating a path to our hotel door.

Back at M&M Products in Atlanta, I immersed myself further into R&D. Emboldened by our success with Sta Sof Fro Regular and Extra Dry Spray, I embarked on developing other products. I was a member of the Society of Cosmetic Chemists because I wanted to know more about current research, as well as the products already on the market, and this membership was useful in my research because it gave me access to people working in the industry, people with whom I could compare notes.

A lot of the company's growth was due to the success of the sprays that Therman and I developed. Therman was particularly good at coming up with ideas, and I was particularly good at developing them. That's how we started with Sta Sof Fro, and that's how we continued to work until the early '80s. Sta Sof Fro Extra Dry had been another of Therman's ideas.

"We should make another Sta Sof Fro brand product," Therman said to me one day in my office. He pointed at the phone on my desk. "The bottle should be the color of that phone, beige."

"What's the difference between Sta Sof Fro and the new product?" I asked, leaning forward in my chair. I loved hashing out ideas, especially with Therman. The feeling was always one of excitement over the prospect of creating something new.

"No difference, really. Same formula, new fragrance. We use new packaging."

"What if we actually have a new product? I've been working on a new formula, using it on myself." I patted my hair. "It has the same softening effect as Sta Sof Fro, but it's better. It contains more conditioners and a new fragrance."

"Well," Therman smiled as he got up. "It looks like we've got our Sta Sof Fro Extra Dry."

We did, and it took off like a rocket. The new, enriched formula with a better fragrance was an improvement on our own product that was already dominating the market. We put our Extra Dry before the competition had a chance to make one of their own, and we reaped the rewards for doing so. That product, which became known as "the product in the beige bottle," launched M&M Products Company beyond our wildest dreams. Sales jumped from $800,000 in 1978, to $8 million in 1979.

In addition, I had my ear to the ground, something that was always a part of putting Sta Sof Fro into people's hands. I talked to stylists and consumers, listening for comments, requests and ideas. It was through the salons that I first learned about the emerging popularity of the curl. Michael Jackson epitomized the look during his "Thriller" period, along with other entertainers such as Prince and Smokey Robinson. It was the many athletes, however, especially basketball players, who helped popularize the curl look.

The curl was a cream-based chemical process of changing the configuration pattern of the hair's curl at the molecular level. First, the hair was straightened. Then, depending on the size of the curl desired, the straightened hair was wrapped around a small, medium, or large rod. The hair then "set" to a loose curl, which lasted up to eight weeks. This curl process allowed people to wear a new style. It was shinier and had looser curls than the Afro, but the chemical process left hair terribly dry. That is where Sta Sof Fro came in as a key element of the curl process.

Jheri Redding was the first to come out with the Jheri Curl, and because he was the first one to start the style, it became known simply as "the Jheri Curl," and later just "the curl." I learned early on through people in the field, such as stylists, that the technicians who developed Jheri Curl had not created any maintenance products to compensate for the dry hair that resulted from the curl process. Instead, they used Sta Sof Fro, and in turn told stylists to use it, too. And so, Sta Sof Fro, originally developed to keep Afros soft, was swept up into this new style. In fact, Sta Sof Fro had actually made these styles possible in the first place, since without it, there would be no saving the dry hair.

Therman and I not only developed curl-maintenance sprays in the Sta Sof Fro line, we had also worked this newfound feature of Sta Sof Fro into our current advertising.

"Let's do more," I suggested to Therman, after meeting with the marketing department. "Let's develop a brand for women. We've got to do more to address the curl market." Around 80 % of our Sta Sof Fro users were men, and the unisex spray was performing well.

Therman smiled. "If we've got to grow, we've got to grow."

I met with our research and development staff, and we eventually came up with the Soft 'n Free brand of curl-maintenance products to cater to women, and to be a broad enough line that could deal with a number of styles. Even though Sta Sof Fro had been instrumental in the curl style, it had been branded as an Afro softener for men. Developing a line with a broader appeal would position M&M to adapt to any emerging styles.

As we worked on developing new Sta Sof Fro and Soft 'n Free curl- maintenance products while marketing those we had recently released, Sta Sof Fro kept flying off the shelves, our maintenance products held steady, and M&M continued to grow like crazy. Once again, sales doubled that year, and M&M products were popular nationwide.

Chapter 16: The Center Does Not Hold

The 1980s are generally known as the "Me Generation," in which "conspicuous consumption" became the norm for most Americans. Focusing their purchase power on material goods benefited companies such as M&M. For my family and my company, however, the decade turned out to be a devastating one. Despite everything that happened over those ten years, I managed to hold on, although there were times when it was not easy.

Through the 1970s, things had been going better than I could have ever imagined, though I was not surprised by the success. After all, I had dreamt of that idea and worked hard for it since I was a child. So at the start of the new decade, between personal and professional successes and new experiences, Therman and I had good reason to be happy. M&M Products' wealth continued to grow and was now a multimillion-dollar company. Once again, we outgrew our offices on Royal Drive, and so Therman and I decided we needed to move. We found 50,000 square feet near our old facilities on Browns Mill Road in 1981. Our executive and administrative offices, along with our shipping department, would now be on Browns Mill Road, while manufacturing would remain on Royal Drive. There was renovating to be done on the offices, but even when they were done, M&M would continue to grow until it occupied more than 300,000 square feet.

With so much to do, I overlooked small clues that my relationship with Therman was beginning to deteriorate. We had always worked side by side, from the assembly line in Therman's basement to our offices at the first Browns Mill Road location and then on Royal Drive. But during the building renovations at our second Browns Mill location, I learned that Therman had decided to have his office suite at the other end of the building. "He wants that corner," Eli told me by way of explanation. I did not give it much thought at first, but eventually it became clear something was not right between Therman and me.

"What's going on with you and Therman?" Mitch McKinney, our sales V.P., asked me shortly after we had moved back to Browns Mill Road. He had just walked down the hall from Therman's newly finished office.

"What are you talking about?"

"Well, he's talking about how frustrated he is with everything. He feels like you've just taken over."

I opened my mouth, but then closed it. Finally, I said, "Well, I'll go see what's going on in a while." I knew I had better confront Therman directly with what I'd heard rather than discuss it with anyone else. It would get back to him just as the comment he supposedly made had got back to me. Any problems we had, I thought, we could work out just between us. Later, I went to see him.

Closing his office door behind me, I asked, "Therman, what is going on? Mitch is telling me you and I have a problem."

He shook his head and shrugged. "No, man, there's no problem." Then he laughed. "You know how some of these guys are. They gossip like women."

I did not pursue it with him further. I believed our relationship was strong. Besides, there was no time to think about it.

At our newest location, we were growing rapidly to 400 employees, hiring more staff, manufacturing and managerial people, working especially hard to plump up our marketing division. There was a lot of time spent organizing and reorganizing the corporate structure because we knew doing so was essential to our future. It wasn't always smooth going, but Therman and I worked to do what was best for the company, and so also what was best for all of us as employees.

We brought in Dr. Josiah Pierson, the former Dean of Students at Fort Valley College, as our new director of human resources, and Bob Hudson became our brand manager, Dick Hearnes came over from rival Johnson Products. Kay Osborne, a politically connected Jamaican with extensive international marketing experience, came aboard as our director of international sales at the recommendation of Atlanta politician Andy Young.

We also lured Fleetwood Price from Coca-Cola after we learned about him through Joyce McGriff.

Unfortunately, Fleetwood lasted only ten months of a lucrative two-year contract.

Fleetwood made a number of changes that did not serve M&M's interests. At his direction, M&M had contracted with a small agency, KK&B, for all our advertising. Though the radio spots were good, they were not realizing much in sales. When sales were anything short of brisk, there was reason to be concerned. Not only this, but the direction we had planned before Fleetwood came on board had been changed. Worse yet, we were paying $24,000 a month to KK&B for this change, and it was not sitting right with me.

Not only did I have questions about initiatives and expenditures such as those in advertising, but I also saw departmental conflict. Fleetwood seemed to rub almost everyone the wrong way. His abrasive style meant numerous run-ins with his colleagues, and the tension created was undermining company camaraderie and unity. He had come in as a take-charge, organizational executive, which was exactly what we wanted, and he had brought needed structure to the marketing department. For that we were grateful, but within six months, it was clear that the changes in the advertising campaigns we had planned were not taking effect. I realized that Therman and I needed to step in. I knew that I, for one, was not feeling Fleetwood anymore.

I decided that I had to talk to Therman about my growing concern that perhaps we had made a mistake in hiring Fleetwood. After missing him several times at the office, I finally got hold of Therman by going straight to his house one weekend. I found him in his yard, raking some leaves.

"Something is just not right," I told him, and laid out everything that had been bothering me about Fleetwood's handling of the marketing department. If I thought I would get support, I was wrong.

"Cornell," Therman responded dismissively, "just back off of him. Leave him be and let him do his job."

"I *am* letting him do his job. That's the problem! Why are you defending him? Doesn't it bother you that we're spending all this money but not seeing any results?"

But Therman and Fleetwood had become close, and this would prove to be one of the factors that eventually drove a wedge between Therman and me. Fleetwood even used Therman in an advertisement for M&M Products as a way of getting into Therman's head. After that, Fleetwood could do no wrong. Therman began to kowtow to Fleetwood, approving everything Fleetwood wanted to do. At the time, however, I knew none of this. I just knew that something was not right.

I decided to turn to Lafayette Jones, whom we hired several years before as a marketing consultant after he had left Johnson Products. Laf first came to my attention when he was V.P. of marketing and sales at Johnson Products. He had also worked for Kraft on such brands as Manwich and Orville Redenbacher, but at Johnson he was in direct competition with M&M. In his capacity there, he tried to derail us, but George Johnson wouldn't let him. Later, Laf told me, "George didn't want to mess with you and Therman 'cause he said you were nice guys. I said, 'Fine, they're nice guys, but we need their market.' I just could not understand why he let you grow and grow." When George Johnson hired Laf, that was the talk of the industry, because of his background with those large white companies like Kraft and General Foods.

So he was a well-known figure in the industry when I finally saw him for the first time when he came to Atlanta to appear on "Ebony Beat Journal." He was still with Johnson at the time, but when asked about M&M, he was very complimentary. I knew then that he was not only a talented marketer, he was also a good politician.

Sometime after he left Johnson, I recruited him as our marketing consultant. It was Laf who had first encouraged us to diversify our Sta Sof line beyond the softener, shampoo and moisturizer, and the continued development of Soft 'n Free was the result. It was, in part, through my education with Laf that I had become a firm believer in expanding M&M. He and I agreed that a single line of products devoted to the male market would not sustain the company.

Though Fleetwood did not like Laf at first, Laf was able to work around him, and in the end they became friendly. Fleetwood was an excellent administrator who could make things happen, but Laf was more creative.

"Something's not right," I told Laf. "And I need your help."

"Mac, you're right. Advertising is a problem. $24,000 a month is too steep," Laf told me shortly after my conversation with Therman. I had asked him to look into M&M's advertising with another one of our marketing people, Dick Hearns, and both he and Dick met with me to discuss their findings.

"I can't see why Bill is charging us that kind of money," said Laf, a hint of doubt creeping into his voice. Bill Sharp was a former Coca-Cola man who went over to KK&B as its president. He and Fleetwood were good friends, and according to Fleetwood, Bill was going to help us gain a foothold in the curl market.

"Fleetwood says Bill is the one to turn things around," I replied.

"That may be true," Laf said, "but not for that kind of money. No way."

"Fifteen is more like it," Dick added.

I sighed, knowing that I had to fix the advertising budget, but not wanting to cause strife between Laf, Dick and Fleetwood. But this was different. Fleetwood and Laf had a tenuous relationship already, and I was sure Fleetwood would resent being told to change the advertising budget based on a conversation he was not in on. I also knew that Therman would be upset if I could not convince him that there was a problem affecting M&M's sales. I valued open, free dialogue as the best way to hash out ideas and solve problems.

I tracked Therman down once again, and explained the situation. "I am concerned," I said. "The money just does not make sense. The ad campaign is not in sync with the market. I mean, what is Fleetwood doing with a guy who is older than the market demographic, and who works for a white agency that has no experience in the black hair-care market. I am telling you, it does not make sense. Come on," I practically pleaded. "We have to work on this together."

He thought about it for a moment before responding. "I don't know," he said hesitantly. He realized that something was not right. "Fleetwood's a friend of mine. I don't want to hurt him. I certainly don't want to change things in midstream and make it seem like I don't back up his decisions."

"I know it, I understand. But I have gone over the figures. We are not getting the most out of what we're spending."

"So maybe it's not the advertising that's the problem. We've had trouble with the curl products from day one."

"That could be, but if advertising is not the problem, if the products just aren't selling, then we have no product to advertise. If the advertising's no good, we are wasting money. If the product is not going to sell better no matter how much we spend on advertising, then why spend the money on advertising? Either way, we're spending too much money."

Therman finally agreed. "Okay, but let's see what they say before we tell them to cut it down. Let's talk to Fleetwood and Bill."

"You're right. Maybe we need to discuss the advertising budget with both of them—with Fleetwood and Bill together—in a relaxed environment, we can sort out the money."

So the four of us—Therman , Fleetwood, Bill and I—had dinner together. Though we were out on business, it felt good to spend time again with Therman.

He and I talked and laughed, enjoying each other for
the first time in a long while. Fleetwood, who was usually not very cordial to me and often even arrogant,
was amiable. Still, as the night wore on, the atmosphere felt increasingly strange, as if Fleetwood and Bill
were merely tolerating the evening.

I said, "Therman and I wanted to discuss the
advertising budget with you."

Bill and Fleetwood glanced at each other. "Well,
sure," Bill said with a tone that sounded to me of false
congeniality. "Why else would the four of us get
together?"

I turned to Fleetwood and asked, "Are we getting
the most for our money?"

"If I didn't think so, I wouldn't be spending it."

"Could you be wrong?"

His eyes narrowed briefly, trying to read my face.
"We could all be wrong."

Soon after that meeting, I heard from one of the
marketing people that Fleetwood was commenting
about me, "I wish he would just get the hell out of my
hair and go fishing."

That angered me. I had worked hard to make sure
that everyone had the freedom, from the bottom up, to
tell me what they thought, and Therman and I had
every right to ask all our executives to account for the
decisions they made. Yes, I was involved in the company, but I always trusted everyone to do their job until
they proved otherwise. Not only that, if Fleetwood felt
I was too intrusive, he should have come to me directly. If he felt that the problem with Soft 'n Free was not
marketing, we could have hashed that out.

In the end, it was apparent to me that M&M Products would have to part ways with KK&B—and with Fleetwood Price. We never did get to the bottom of the Fleetwood issue, and Therman and I finally agreed to let Fleetwood go. Fortunately for us, we had Kay Osborne, who was in charge of international sales, and was doing a terrific job. Therman and I agreed to make her V.P. of marketing after Fleetwood's departure. She quickly organized the department, rallying the troops in sales with motivational field visits and an overall sense that everyone's contribution to the company mattered. Kay had a tremendous amount of energy and knowledge to help get us back on track, and she worked day and night to revitalize the department, broaden the Soft 'n Free brand, and pull everyone together in a spirit of unity.

Seeking out and hiring people we thought would excel in their positions, and thereby help M&M grow, had been a wonderful, if sometimes nerve-wracking opportunity. It was a way of building up our community, and we were generous employers. Our salary structure was considered the best in the industry, with top employees averaging $100,00 a year—an impressive amount in any era, but certainly in the 1980s—and a benefits package that equaled giant soft drink company, Coca-Cola. Our salary motto was, "We pay higher than the industry." Therman and I believed in paying well because we valued our employees' contributions to the success of the company, and paying well was one of the ways we were able to bring in terrific talent.

One of the high points of M&M Products growth

and development was in 1981. We had promoted each of our department managers to the title, Vice President, and looked forward to a bright future. We had achieved $30 million in sales, and as a reward to the sales department, we took the entire sales force to Acapulco for our annual sales meeting—all expenses paid, and no expense spared. It was first class all the way. We stayed at the Princess, whose employees referred to us as "the rich black Americans." That $250,000 trip became legendary in the industry, and people still talk about it today.

I sent the marketing department into the field, MBAs who had loads of theory but no practical experience with selling, and so ideas that did not incorporate all-important field knowledge. Even managers had to go work on the line, and I put myself there, too. I spent time in the warehouses and on the assembly. (I wasn't surprised when, a number of years later, a business book entitled, *Managing By Walking Around* came out. The moment I saw it, everything I had been doing crystallized in my mind. Oh, I thought. So *that's* what I was doing!)

The more the managers and executives knew about practice, the better informed their proposals would be. On my side, the more I learned from them about theory, about the logic behind their thinking, the better able I would be to make decisions that affected the direction of the company.

I was relentless. "Talk to me," I would say to people as I entered their department. "Give me the options." I learned to listen and encouraged discussion. I wanted active brains, not brains neutralized by bosses who dictated to them and stifled thinking. This was a crucial moment for me. I had overcome my own insecurity and adjusted to the new circumstances. But that adjustment did not work for everyone.

After much effort, our corporate structuring was complete, and I was confident in my role. M&M Products was now positioned to become one of the most successful black-owned companies in America. *Black Enterprise* magazine named M&M Products the 11th largest black-owned company, and we were consistently on their list throughout the 1980s. *Jet* magazine ran a story about the wonderful actress, Esther Rolle, who was a fan of Sta Sof Fro. In that article, she spoke of her fondness for the product. The matriarch of the popular television comedy, *Good Times*, had a fantastic Afro, and was friendly with one of M&M's marketing people, and we were fortunate to get to know her. We hosted her at the company offices when she visited Atlanta, and she kindly welcomed my family when we visited Los Angeles on vacation.

In business and in the community, Therman and I were well respected. We were also well known. *Ebony* magazine did a feature story on Therman and me, and we were regularly interviewed for local television programs and news stories. Part of our popularity was due to the success of the business, but also to our charitable giving, such as educational scholarships and donations to community organizations.

M&M Products' Community Relations department had an extensive budget, and I was proud of our philanthropic endeavors and my involvement in local politics. Along with this success came new opportunities.

I was offered, and accepted, a number of board appointments, including the National Bank of Georgia, the Atlanta Chamber of Commerce and the Atlanta Symphony.

I was one of the founding members of the American Health and Beauty Aids Institute (AHBAI), which was started by Lafayette Jones and Grayson Mitchell in 1981. The AHBAI was established as a trade association, a marketing tool that would get our products into more stores. Many large chains, such as Walgreens and K-mart, stocked products according to residence demographics. So if a neighborhood was predominantly white, the local K-mart would not stock so-called ethnic hair care and other products. With the strength of the AHBAI membership, chains were persuaded to rethink their position. Just because a neighborhood's residence had a certain racial demographic did not mean that no one else ever visited their stores. Black people, we argued, do not just shop where they live anymore than white people do. They also shop where they work. In the end, AHBAI was effective in increasing distribution of our company's various products, and a number of chains began selling our products in all their stores.

My interest in distribution was not limited to large retail chains. I thought M&M should invest in its own stores, so that we could control our distribution. It seemed clear to me that if we established our own beauty supply stores nationwide, we could prevent the competition from monopolizing the market on product distribution. Beauty supply retailers made more than a tidy profit on both sides—the consumer paid a high price for products, and the distributor bought from the manufacturer at a fairly low price. I also thought it was just a matter of time before the beauty supplier would control the market and thus the manufacturer. Why not, I wondered, cut out the distributor and put M&M and other similar companies in his place?

Few people, unfortunately, were ultimately interested, including my colleagues at the AHBAI, and my partner, Therman. "Why do we need to get into distribution?" Therman asked me. "We have everything we need right here."

I had walked down the hall to his office for a chat, where I discussed some ideas I had about the direction we should head in the coming years. Among the things I was thinking about was distribution. "The question is, why *shouldn't* we get into distribution," I responded. "There is no reason why we should not have outlets to sell directly to customers. We're all over the country now, in big outlets like K-Mart—"

"Exactly," Therman interrupted. "And it's working fine."

"For now. But when sales start to get squeezed, it would be good to have stores in place that we own."

"Cornell, as long as people have got hair on their heads, they will need Sta Sof Fro."

I protested, but Therman did not want any part of it. He believed things were fine the way they were. From my field experience, reading various sources across the industry, such as *Advertising Age* and other trade publications, and through my associations with AHBAI, it was clear to me that the industry was in a period of change. When I looked to the future, I saw a formerly black-owned and- operated industry losing the distribution side of the "ethnic" products business. Many black-owned beauty and barber-supply stores were being bought up, and so I made several more attempts to convince Therman that M&M should own its own distribution centers.

"Man, look at the figures," I pleaded. "Within the next ten years, things will change and I do not want to be held hostage by Sally's or the Koreans, who are going to dominate distribution if we don't get in on it. We can do something about it before it's too late."

"Uh-huh," he shook his head. "I don't see it. We make the product. That's good enough for me."

I was frustrated. It was our first real impasse about the future of our company. "I guarantee you, owning distribution is going to be important. Look at Sally's. They've got less than 50 stores now, but I will bet you they will be all over the country in the next 10 to 15 years." Sally's Beauty Supply was just getting started, and it was true that by the end of the 1990s they would have more than 2,000 stores nationwide. The Koreans were beginning to enter the distribution market in a big way, and I saw the writing on the wall. Once they had a virtual monopoly on distribution, they'd set the prices, and they would come out on top. "Therman, listen to me. You and I, and M&M, have got to keep diversifying, and we have to hold on to this market." When all was said and done, I undertook diversification on my own, with the hope that my projects could be later incorporated into M&M.

In the meantime, I involved myself further in R&D,

hiring cosmetic chemist James Agard away from Estée Lauder to work with Eli in research and development. Though the maintenance products were doing well overall, there were some product performance issues that needed to be addressed.

In 1981 we had put out our first chemical curl line under the Soft 'n Free brand, Soft 'n Free Chemical Curl kit. We started developing it in the late '70s, after other chemical-curl products had already established themselves. The success of Sta Sof Fro, and Soft 'n Free maintenance products in the curl market encouraged us to try competing with established products such as Jheri Curl and Care Free Curl by Soft Sheen out of Chicago. Soft Sheen was already doing big sales numbers by the time we decided to get into the curl market with new products. Though we were late getting into the race, R&D was adamant about the superiority of our brand.

"It's better for the hair," Eli said at the time. "People will see the difference."

"Well," I responded, "we've got to have *something* to bring customers over to us. These other guys have entire lines devoted to the curl. Until now, we've just had the maintenance products." Customers tended to buy within a brand. So, whatever brand they used to create the curl, they used the same one to maintain the style. One brand's shampoos, conditioners and sprays all worked to support the brand's chemical. So, if customers used Carefree Curl, for example, they looked for Carefree Curl maintenance products.

While we worked to market our chemical and maintenance products in 1981 and 1982, I also moved from department to department to help where needed. Even though our team was complete, and every department was fully staffed with experts in their fields, I wanted to keep abreast of what was going on, offer advice and learn from everyone.

In 1982, while waiting to see if the chemical-curl products would gain a foothold in the curl market, I opened the first of ten beauty supply stores around Atlanta, White's Discount Beauty Center, and asked an old friend from Savannah, Calvin O'Neill, to oversee operations. My family also got involved in White's, too. With Cornell Jr. about to go to college and having grown up helping on the basement assembly line, it seemed natural for him to come into the family business when he graduated. Sheila was getting close to graduation, and I hoped that she would want to get involved, too. Sholanda, and little André, who was just 6, already helped out at White's after school. André would ring up sales and then return to the floor to play with his toy trucks, and Sholanda would help direct customers to the products they wanted. Harriet was there every day, making sure the store was running smoothly.

As part of my diversification plan that I hoped eventually to bring M&M into, I also opened a liquor store called Jolly Mac's that I hoped to build into a chain. An old friend from Savannah, who had run a bar there, came up to manage it.

It felt good to be able to create businesses because I was providing jobs. Of course, I had started that process with M&M. There, employees had generous salaries and benefits packages, and it delighted me to again provide opportunities to people who just needed a leg up. I suppose that desire to help others came from my belief that when you succeed, you have an obligation to help others. I did not want to be a black man who made it, and then forgot from whence he came.

In the meantime at M&M, problems with the chemical curl were becoming apparent. There were two problems, actually, and as I thought about what was wrong with our chemical-curl product sales, it became obvious to me those two problems were related.

One problem was that the successful brands had cream-based curl chemical products. Another problem was that the hair relaxers were also cream-based formulations, and the salons were familiar with those cream products. Naturally, when the curl came along, stylists gravitated toward the cream products. Consumers also reached for cream products when they went to the store. Our product was liquid-based, and all of the established and best-selling chemical products were cream-based. We never considered this a problem until the product did not sell. People are creatures of habit, and hair product users are no different. Just as they reach for the same brand time after time, they also look for essentially the same product across brands—in the case of the chemical curl, they looked for cream.

At first, we had said, "everyone else had a cream, but we have a liquid. Ours is better." But it wasn't better to have no sales, and Soft 'n Free Curl was not selling.

When I brought it up at our next R&D meeting, suggesting we move to a cream-based curl, Eli and

Therman balked. M&M's Education Department, led by Jim Williams, had been particularly opposed to changing the liquid system.

"We don't have the equipment for it," Therman said, as if it was ridiculous even to consider putting out a chemical-curl product. All our equipment was designed to manufacture liquid products, not creams. It had become apparent that the equipment was a major problem, but when we started the products, we thought everything was fine.

"Besides," Eli continued, "I think it's not the product, it's the people selling it. The sales department isn't doing a good enough job. Why aren't we talking to them?"

"We *are* talking to them," I said. "But that's not the source of the problem. The product is."

"It's fine the way it is," Therman said. "The products will come around, and if they don't, we've got the Sta Sof Fro maintenance products, anyway." Then he added, "You've got your Soft 'n Free Curl Moisturizing Spray, too, so what's the problem?"

My Soft 'n Free? I thought incredulously. Though I never considered it my brand—everything I did was always for M&M, not myself—I had come up with the curl-maintenance product, Soft 'n Free Curl Moisturizing Spray. I shook my head. "Therman, we've got to have the chemical *and* the maintenance line. They go together. Sales of the maintenance products will increase if we have the chemical, too."

Worse still, our product just did not have the ease of use that creams did. With cream chemicals, all you had to do was put the curl cream on the hair, cover it with a plastic cap, wait for the desired straightness, and then rinse it out. Soft 'n Free Chemical Curl had about six steps too many—and it wasn't a cream. Soft Sheen's Carefree Curl home kit had only two steps. Worse yet, our product tended to drip rather than stay on the hair like the creams did.

I shook my head. "We should have gotten the equipment to manufacture creams, or at least contracted out to a lab that could handle it. It would have been in the Sta Sof tradition, but in a more manageable form. People don't want products that run." I was frustrated. Dr. Eli McKenzie was an excellent chemist in his area, and had set up manufacturing beautifully, but had no background in product formulation. He did not know about cosmetic chemistry.

"We were fine with Sta Sof Fro," Therman muttered.

"Look, it was a misstep. No doubt about that. But let's hash this out and get our footing back. If we know where we went wrong, and we can change course, we can fix it." I looked around the room. "I'm going back out into the street. I'm going to talk to people. You should do the same."

Eli spoke again, his voice strained. "I—we put in a lot of time into this. It is a superior product." His team nodded, backing him up.

"It is a superior product, you are right," I agreed. "It is a superior product that is sitting on the shelves. If it isn't selling, we can't pretend it is superior. Why did we not nip this in the bud?" I asked as much to myself as to them. "If what is best for the hair does not sell, then it is not doing anyone's hair any good." We did not have repeat sales, which is confirmation of a product's quality. By the mid-80s, after trying to play catch-up with the curl market, we had to rethink what we were doing.

I became so engrossed in every department of M&M in an effort to reverse the curl debacle, and to set a development and branding course that would take us into the 1990s, that I did not notice the ground giving way beneath my feet. More clues surfaced that distance was growing between Therman and me.

But even with those clues, I wasn't catching on. It was not until Harriet expressed concern that I really took notice. I came home from work one Friday evening to find that Harriet was not ready for a company party at Therman's house. "What's going on? Are you feeling okay?" I asked. "We have to be at Therman's in an hour."

"I don't want to go," she said.

"What? Why?"

"You don't see it, Cornell, but I do."

I was lost. "See what?"

"Therman. Things have changed, Cornell. Therman doesn't treat you right."

Her comment stunned me. I hadn't noticed anything different since the day Therman and I met at Fort Valley College in 1967. But I could not ignore what Harriet was saying.

"He is jealous, or angry—I don't know. I do know that something is not right between you."

"Harriet, why? This is out of the blue—"

"It is not out of the blue," she interrupted. "Think about it. You are the face of the company. When a magazine wants an interview, who do they call? You. Then your board appointments and political involvement. "

This time, I interrupted her. "It is not me alone.

M&M is both of us. Therman has never been interested in those things. He supports them, for sure, but you know him. He never wanted all that."

"Maybe not. But I have noticed a difference. Didn't you ever wonder why, when you moved back over to the new Browns Mill Road location, your offices weren't next to each other anymore? You have been running with a different crowd for a few years now. You get all the attention. I think he realized a while ago that he wanted it."

"Well, then why didn't he just say so? We always shared everything." I was at a loss. "What do I do now?" I asked, half to myself, and half to Harriet.

We went to the party anyway. It would have been unseemly not to go. I spent the entire time watching Therman, trying to pick up signals that something was wrong. I could not put my finger on it then, and not later, either, but there was an air that things were not right. Small things happened at the party, which, once I saw them, I realized had been going on for some time. People came to talk to me, and Therman hung back, quiet most of the time. When he did speak that night, there were other signals.

As Therman and several others and I stood chatting, one of our sales people approached: "Mr. McKenzie, I have people already asking about the next product in the Soft 'n Free line. I think things are turning around for the line," she said optimistically.

"Yeah, well, that's Mr. McBride's product. You'll have to talk to him about it."

"Therman," I laughed uneasily, "what do you mean, 'my product'? It's all M&M, man. It's a way to broaden the company, not me."

As Harriet and I drove home that night, I realized there was much about my relationship with Therman I had not noticed. Maybe I had not wanted to, but it was there. I sighed loud enough for Harriet to hear me.

"I told you," she said.

"Maybe he needs to have more of a public face," I mused. I had to think of something that would make Therman feel less marginalized. I decided to work harder at making sure I was not the sole face of M&M Products. Later, around 1983 and 1984, when I was offered more board appointments, even when Governor Joe Frank Harris's office called to ask, I declined them. Besides, I figured that there was so much going on already, I did not need further distractions from the business.

I resolved to talk to him the following Monday, after a sales meeting scheduled first thing in the morning. But when I sat down in the conference room, there was no Therman. I picked up a phone and called over to his office. His secretary answered.

"Sorry, Mr. McBride," she said. "I reminded him about this morning's meeting, but he said he was out in the field and he would call you later."

"All right," I replied, and hung up. I was confused, and decided to reschedule the meeting for another time. I caught him later that day in his office.

"Hey man," I said as I walked into his office. "We missed you this morning."

"Oh," he said vaguely, flipping through papers on his desk. "I had to miss the meeting."

"Yeah, I know." I sat down in the chair opposite his

desk. After he did not saying anything more, I continued. "Well, we have to reschedule. Sales needs some
direction. Have you talked to the guys in shipping
lately? They tell me that they have back orders, but
management has not taken care of it."

Therman only shrugged, seemingly disinterested
in what I had to say. "Therman, what is going *on*?"

"What do you mean?" He kept his eyes on the
papers in front of him.

"I think you're upset with me."

This seemed to startle him, and he looked up and
gave a short laugh. "No, man. I'm not mad at you.
We're good."

"You sure?"

"Yeah, I'm sure."

"All right, then," I said, getting up. "I'll talk to
you." If he did not want to talk about it, then I was not
going to push him. Instead, I decided to try another
way. As I walked toward the door, I said, "There's a
fund-raiser for Andy Young's candidacy this week.
Why don't you come with me to that? I miss seeing
you, Therman." I paused at the door.

Andrew Young had recently returned to Atlanta
after serving as ambassador to the United Nations
during Jimmy Carter's presidency. Now Andy was
running for mayor, and I was involved in raising
money for his campaign. Though Therman had
expressed admiration for Andy in the past, he had
never accepted an offer to get involved.

This time, however, to my relief he said yes.
"Good," I said. "That is good news."

Once Therman got involved, he was bitten by the politics bug. At the fundraiser, Therman wanted to donate $10,000. "No, man," I said, "no one is giving more than $500."

"All right, let's give a thousand." Just as he was generous with a dollar in his charitable dealings, so he was with political donations.

Soon enough, Therman was so involved with the Young campaign and other political organizations, he began to miss meetings regularly. They either had to be rescheduled, or if that was not possible, I had to fill him in when he did show up. We were used to talking two and three times a day, and that had changed before I introduced him to politics, but now I was lucky if I spoke with him once a week. Whenever I called over, he was out of the office, or his secretary said he was too busy to talk. Still, when I did speak with him, he insisted everything between us was okay. I tried everything I could think of, including suggesting that his title be changed to "Chairman," which he wanted. But nothing seemed to work.

I was worried. Therman and I had been a team. Our collective strength was how our individual strengths complemented each other. Now, since we hardly saw each other, the company was getting mixed signals. Sometimes I did not know what Therman told one department, and then I would say almost the opposite. Since we were hardly talking, there was no discussion and so no compromise. The marketing department especially began to feel pulled in too many directions.

One of those directions was the advertising and

marketing of Natural Light. "You have Soft 'n Free, I have Natural Light," Therman declared after I found out he was putting out another product under the Sta Sof Fro brand. Therman began developing Natural Light soon after M&M came out with Soft 'n Free— before Soft 'n Free could get off the ground and contribute to sales. Because I had developed Soft 'n Free, Therman began to think of it as "mine." Though I never thought that, it was in his head, and the result was Natural Light.

"How many times do I have to tell you that Soft 'n Free is not mine?"

"I've already got Andy committed to a few spots—"

"Andy? Andy *Young*?" I was stunned. We had discussed none of this.

"Yeah, that's right. Andy Young. He's got that great Afro—is that a problem?" he challenged me.

I was speechless. Not only had he got Andy to endorse the product, he insisted on sharing advertising dollars between the two brands, and in doing that, undermined any possibility for success. Money taken away from Soft 'n Free, which was already on the market, meant that its sales would drop.

"Therman, Soft 'n Free is just starting to gain a foothold. We need to put our advertising efforts in that direction."

"Listen, you do your thing, and I will do mine." With that, he walked away from me. Unfortunately for M&M and Soft 'n Free, Natural Light was a disaster.

The company needed both of us, and needed unity. I knew I had to double my involvement in every aspect of M&M. I went to every department meeting, not just the regularly scheduled meetings of all our vice presidents. In order to mitigate some of the disorganization that resulted from Therman and my lack of communication, I wanted to know how individual departments were running. I also wanted to gauge their internal structure—how they were being managed by their VPs. Through the mid-80s we're still struggling in the curl market after our initial failure, and it was not going to get much better. In fact, my family and I had already been dealing with problems of our own.

Chapter 17: Disintegration

"What is Chronic Nephritic Syndrome?" I asked the doctor.

Sheila, Harriet and I sat in the doctor's office—the fourth we had seen since Sheila first began feeling sick in 1982. It had started with her complaining that her feet and ankles were swelling. "How can I be getting fat in my *feet*?" she had asked. But then her legs swelled up, and before long, she was swollen even around her eyes. At the same time, she was having trouble breathing and always felt weak. Right then we knew we needed to get to the bottom of these strange symptoms. At 20 years old, Sheila should be beginning her adult life, not feeling so sick and weak, and having a body so swollen that she could not function like the normal, vibrant young woman she had been all her life.

After several misdiagnoses, we finally found a doctor who got it right. "Chronic Nephritic Syndrome is a condition in which there are high levels of protein in the urine, high cholesterol and the sort of swelling that Sheila has been experiencing. All this is caused by damage to the kidney's blood vessels, which means the kidneys don't filter waste properly. There are a number of possible causes. In young children, it is very often treated successfully, and the type of treatment depends on the underlying cause. In adults, however, it's much trickier. It may be incurable."

"Incurable?" I asked. Harriet and I exchanged stricken glances.

The doctor went on matter-of-factly. "Most likely, yes. But not unmanageable. It is imperative that Sheila begins treatment right away, because, as I said, Sheila's kidneys are not properly filtering fluids. As a result, she is losing large quantities of protein—there is a lot in her urine, but very low levels in her blood."

"She's not a child, but she is so young," I pleaded. "She could still be okay, couldn't she?"

"It is a rare disease. As I said, it's a condition she'll have to adjust to, not get over. Diabetes is the most common cause in adults. Lupus is also a cause. Sometimes, we cannot find the cause at all, but I still need to run more tests."

"But we can start helping her now, right?" I asked, feeling both increasingly helpless and determined to do whatever it took to make my daughter well again.

"Yes, we can start now with prednisone—that's a steroid. But we also have to make sure Sheila, and you, are educated about how the disease and the medications affect the body."

Harriet listened to all this patiently, but there was pain in her eyes. She sat next to a listless Sheila, occasionally reaching over to pat her daughter's hand. It would be Harriet who bore the burden of Sheila's care. As things were beginning to unravel at M&M, I found myself putting in the sort of hours as Therman and I had done at the very beginning. As a result, Harriet was the one who shuttled Sheila to her doctors appointments, oversaw her diet, and generally took care of her while also looking after Sholanda and André and putting in time at our new beauty supply venture.

Still, I wanted to make sure that my daughter received the finest care. Through a physician-friend of mine I was able to get an appointment at Emory University Hospital with one of the finest doctors in the field. He put her on a treatment regime, and Sheila tried her best to live a normal, independent life. She took her medications as directed, but for the next five years, her health continued to decline, and she was in and out of the hospital to receive blood transfusions. Every time she went in, she would come out well, but that never lasted very long.

In the meantime, I put my energies into M&M. That November, I was in Savannah on business. As I did whenever I was there, I went to my parents' new house to check in on them and say hello.

My mother had decorated the house I built her in 1981 with the best of everything, inside and out. Once the construction was nearing completion, I took her shopping for all new furniture and interiors like drapes. She knew exactly what she wanted! She even had her initials, T.M., painted on the awnings she had installed on the windows. Best of all, there was, for the first time in my parents' lives, central air conditioning.

The quaint but large brick house was situated on

property close to the house they used to live in, in an area called Hudson Hill. My siblings and I, at youngest brother, Richard's urging, had pooled our resources and bought them a home nearby some years before. But I had a promise to keep, and a quaint house to build. They had enough room for my dad's dogs and a nice garden, though he had never put one in, and they were close to the Savannah River, where they often fished.

Best of all, my sister Bernice lived with her children right up the street, in a house I had bought for her. Though our parents were self-sufficient, it was nice to have her close by, and her children were constantly at their grandparents' house. They were very close.

When I arrived for my visit, my mother greeted me at the kitchen door.

"Come on inside. I have some hot coffee just brewed."

I kissed her on the cheek. "Thanks, Mom. It's good to see you."

She turned and went into the house, asking about Sheila. "How is she holding up?"

"Well, she is not happy about it, that's for sure. But she's doing all right. It's hard on her. And Harriet."

She shook her head sadly as she moved about the kitchen preparing a snack for us. "That poor girl. Just 20 years old, at the start of her life, and she has this to deal with. A young girl like that is supposed to be out sowing her oats."

"Well," I tried to be light, "she is doing the best she can with the oats she has." I had to be positive or the grief I felt for my first child would swallow me up.

Once we were settled at the kitchen table, we

caught up on the goings-on in the neighborhood. I noticed that the house seemed unusually still. "Say, Mom, where is Dad?" I saw the dogs in the yard, so I knew he was not out hunting.

"Oh, he's in bed. He hasn't been feeling well, lately. You know he's having a rough time." Several of my dad's close friends had recently died, and their passing had been hard on him.

"In bed? In the afternoon?" No matter what, my father was always up in the morning, doing something. "Let me see him."

"All right, but tread lightly with him. He lost another one of his hunting buddies only a short while ago. Heart attack."

"That's too bad. Has he been out since?"

She shook her head. "No. He's almost always in bed since then."

We walked down the hall to my parents' bedroom. My father lay there, surrounded by white sheets and an expanse of homemade quilting. He had always been larger than life to my eyes, but suddenly, despite still weighing in at a solid 230 pounds, he looked frail. "Hey, Daddy," I said quietly leaning over him. "How are you doing?"

His eyelids fluttered. "Cornell?"

"Yes, it's me, Dad."

He reached a shaky hand out from under the covers and acknowledged me. "It is good to see you, son." The last time I saw him he looked well and strong. Now, he looked much older than his 73 years.

"Well, I was down this way, and thought maybe I'd stop in and say hello. You feeling all right?"

He shook his head slightly, closing his eyes. "There's another gone, now. I'm losing them all. Who will I hunt with how?" He swallowed, and then opened his eyes up to me. "You want to do a little hunting?"

I wanted to cheer him up, and though feeling pressed for time, I said, "Sure, dad. That is a nice idea."

Suddenly, his eyes lit up. I looked back at my mother, who stood in the doorway, and smiled. "Mom, Dad and I are going to do a little hunting. What do you say?"

She smiled, and said, "Let me get you something to wear. You can't go out in that nice suit. I think I have another pair of boots around here somewhere, too. Why don't you help my Old Man out of bed, and I'll get you two something to wear. Suddenly finding a reserve of vigor, my father did not need much help out of bed. Mother returned shortly with pants, jackets and two pairs of boots for my dad and me.

Dad sat on the bed once he was dressed, and started pulling on his boots. I threw on his extra pair of camouflage pants and jacket. They hung off me like I was a small child playing dress-up in his father's clothes. My dress shoes jutted out like two buttons from the stiff, boxy pants. "Ready?" I asked, turning to face him.

He was still straining to lace up his boots, coughing each time he leaned forward. "Here," I said, kneeling before him. "I can get those."

Mother sent us off with a wave, and we headed to Dad's truck. The dogs leapt and spun, happy to be heading out on an adventure after so long. Dad's eyes shone behind the dullness I had first seen when he was in bed.

We drove out with the dogs to Five Mile Bend. Once we started walking, though, my dad had trouble breathing. After about a hundred yards, he had to stop. Coughing and wheezing, he struggled for breath.

"Dad," I said urgently, taking his arm. "I've got you. I'm right here."

He nodded, unable to speak. After a while, he said hoarsely, "Okay, now," and patted me on the arm.

We set off again, but it was not long before he began coughing and wheezing once again. "Why don't we rest a while," I suggested, holding his arm once again. I wrapped my other arm around him for more support. After he regained his breath, I asked, "Dad, when was the last time you had a physical?"

He waved off the question. "You can't get to see any doctor these days. It's too hard to get an appointment."

"I'll get one for you. This is one bad, bad cold. We have to get you looked at."

He agreed, and we headed back to the house, where I called an attorney friend of mine who lived in Savannah. It was so long since I lived there that I no longer knew who to go see.

We got to see a doctor that afternoon, who treated Dad for his cold symptoms. "He needs a full physical," I urged the doctor. "Something's not right." Though I was busy with M&M and worrying over my daughter's condition, I was never too busy for my other loved ones, and my insistence that Dad see a doctor would turn out to be life saving.

"All right," the doctor said as he hurried off to his next appointment. "Let the front desk know, and they'll get you in as soon as there's an opening."

That opening was not until January. When I protested, my father stopped me. "Stop your worrying. I'll be fine. It's just a cold."

"You must go to that appointment," I told my parents when I left to fly back to Atlanta. In the meantime, my dad's cold did not go away.

"It's cancer," my mother told me over the phone in January of 1983. "The doctor took x-rays. He wants to send us to an oncologist, a cancer specialist." She tried to play it down, but the news was devastating. The cancer had already spread to his neck and jaws. "What can be done?" I asked. It looked hopeless. "Can we do anything?"

The oncologist said my father was strong enough for surgery. After that, there would be radiation. After that, we would just have to wait and see.

While Mom tended to Dad, I called my brothers and sisters to discuss the news. "We need to come together," I said. "We need to help them through this." Fortunately, there was Bernice around the corner, and most of my other siblings still lived in Savannah. Mom was still in good health and so able to care for Dad throughout his illness.

After his surgery, my father went home. Slowly, he gained some strength, but it wasn't long before the radiation was started. He was exhausted, his skin burned from the heat of the radiation, but he kept at it.

"How would you like to get out in a garden when

all this is over?" I asked him one weekend, as I brought him some coffee. He had loved it so when I was a child, and talked about it often after the mule incident so many years earlier. There I was, a man of 40, with that vision seared into my memory for more than 30 years.

"A garden," he said sleepily.

I bought the property next to my parents' house, and had it plowed. Then I drove down from Atlanta on a Friday night with a hand tiller and garden materials. The next morning after coffee, I headed outside. Around mid-morning, my father, bundled in warm clothing and blankets, pulled up a lawn chair and watched silently from the sidelines. I worked all day Saturday tilling and creating rows. Then I planted seeds and various plants. Every so often, I stopped to wipe my brow and sneak a look at my father, who sat with a loving gaze cast across the neat rows. Not a word was spoken. I knew I had to do something to fill the void he had experienced after losing his close friends, and confronting his own illness.

At the end of the day, I was tired, but felt good. Although I had kept in shape since my Air Force days, going to the gym religiously at least three times a week, there was something particularly fine about cultivating land. It was a feeling similar to creating and growing a beloved business. "Well, Dad, what do you think?"

"Yes," he said in a deep rumble, absorbing every inch with his eyes. "It's fine, fine." He was pleased, and when he became stronger, he took to that garden like a duck to water. It seemed to give him a strength he had lost years ago. He worked that garden every day for five years until he could no longer stand up on his own.

My mother would watch him from the kitchen window, sweet face smiling in that way that made you believe, when you were a child, that your parents knew everything there was to know. "Yes," she said to no one in particular. "You do what you can."

For a while, my father did extraordinarily well, especially given how bad things were when he was diagnosed. Still, the fact of his illness stayed with me always, as did Sheila's.

She was still doing mostly okay on her medications, but was continuously forced in and out of the hospital as her kidneys got worse and worse. Medications managed to slow the disease down, but they never stopped it. She just could not have a regular life.

The worries in my personal life seemed to grow in proportion to my worries at M&M as 1983 turned into 1984. The tension there increased, but I did not know how to diffuse it. To make things worse, our sales projections for 1984 were $60 million, and we spent on marketing and advertising accordingly. But as the year neared an end, it was becoming obvious that we would fall short of those figures. The year 1984 would be our first year of financial loss—about $3 million.

"You've got to cut something," Paul Turner, our V.P. of finance said flatly during a meeting with Therman and me. "Scale down production, advertising, but something."

"Cutting means we lose people," I protested. "If not immediately, then in the future." I could not fathom having to let anyone go.

"Right," Therman said, in what had become a rare moment of agreement. "It's not their fault the curl products aren't doing better." Soft 'n Free, the curl product I created for women, was gaining some of the ground we had lost originally, but it would never take the majority of the market. Therman's product, Natural Light, had not faired even that well.

"If you don't cut something now, I guarantee you, the bank's going to start making you. You are winners now, but even one small step, and they're all over you."

"After all the success we've had?" Therman asked rhetorically. He knew it was true, but was frustrated nonetheless.

"Let me see what options the departments can give us," I offered. "Then we can go from there." I knew I needed to do some thinking. The ride had been fast and smooth, but now there were bumps, and I had to do my part to smooth them out. Eventually, we had to lay off a number of people toward the end of 1984.

Just when things were going badly, they got worse. In the early morning hours of January 14, 1985, I got a call from our facilities manager. "Mr. McBride, there's been an explosion in manufacturing."

"What!" I shot bolt upright in bed, startling Harriet out of sleep.

"It's gone, sir. Completely engulfed in flames."

"Is everyone okay?" I asked helplessly. Since we'd

increased manufacturing shifts, there were people working at all hours of the night.

"Everyone's fine, Mr. McBride. No one's hurt."

I did not have time to sigh in relief. I leaped out of bed and raced to Royal Drive. Therman arrived almost at the same time.

"This can't be happening," I said in disbelief as we watched the building burn. "This cannot be happening."

Chapter 18: The End of An Era

The beginning of 1985 saw our production facilities practically devastated. In order to keep our production schedule on track for our ten product lines, we set up an interim manufacturing line at a nearby facility whose equipment normally handled only three lines. There was no question in our minds that we had to keep production up, not only to stay aggressive in the market by meeting our distributor commitments and keeping products on the shelves, but also to ensure that our employees would not be out of work. We had enough inventory to meet our distribution obligations for about six weeks, but we knew we could not lapse on production, because it would eventually catch up to us.

If the fire at the manufacturing building was not bad enough in 1984, I had a whole basket of problems to choose from. There was M&M's first-ever profit loss to the tune of $3 million. The bank started tightening up on credit right away, as if the preceding ten years of phenomenal success had meant nothing. For the first time we were pressured to cut expenses, which I hated. Previously, Therman and I dealt with obstacles by increasing and by expanding, not by cutting back. Increasingly in the mid-1980s, business was about defense, not offense.

Though in retrospect we were overstaffed, a defensive move like downsizing was emotionally devastating to contemplate. I felt personally responsible for M&M employees. For example, we hired a man who had been on death row, but was released after he was exonerated. When he could not find a job, he was put in contact with M&M, and we found a place for him.

Even when job performance was consistently poor, I preferred trying to help employees turn things around, rather than fire them. This was also the case with my side businesses, Jolly Mack Liquor and White's Discount Beauty Supply. Both businesses were floundering.

"Inventory's walking right out the door, Dad," Cornell Jr. told me. He was finishing up at Howard University, with plans to run the businesses when he graduated. In the meantime, he worked part time. "People see a case of wine and think nothing of taking home a bottle for the evening's entertainment."

He was right. I had hired people who thought nothing of taking whole cases of wine home with them at night. It became a free for all. It was not as simple as I thought it would be to give people an opportunity to succeed. If I had learned anything and taught my children the same, it was that you make sure you know where every last item of inventory is. Unfortunately, the people I had hired did not learn the same. This was also true at White's. When Cornell Jr. did graduate from college, he tried to turn the businesses around. We downsized from ten White's locations to five, put in a computer tracking system in both businesses for accurate inventory, but employees found a way around it and we still lost money.

Of all the professional difficulties I faced that year, however, the worst was the tension that had been building between Therman and me. I kept trying to figure out what I was doing wrong and fix it, but nothing seemed to work. This was especially frustrating to me, since I always believed strongly in assessing and evaluating problems and then doing whatever was necessary to fix them.

Though there was a rupture between us, we saw so little of each other that the division was not obvious to anyone who did not already know about it. Therman had readily taken to Atlanta's political scene and was enthusiastically involved in M&M philanthropic activities. In addition to his deepening interest in politics, Therman accepted a number of board appointments. If he was away from the office a lot before, now he was rarely seen. Without my partner around, it was difficult to run the business effectively. Though surrounded by a number of top-notch executives, Therman was my best friend and confidant. We always used each other as sounding boards, and in his absence, my voice trailed off into thin air.

We were losing money not only in sales, but also in other areas of the company. Many people were overpaid, which would not have been a problem if the company was as healthy as it could be. But if you want to ride on the wagon of success, you had better be willing to get off and pull when you have to. Unfortunately, that was not happening. Things in marketing, for example, were in disarray. The department and I were never in agreement about how to promote Soft 'n Free so that it would be protected from the competition. In addition, the money that we spent on advertising seemed to be giving us diminishing returns. We were marketing a total of 77 products under three brand names, and we could not afford to be weak in any area.

Within the next few years, as we tried to turn things around at M&M, new problems emerged. We were losing good people. Kay Osborne left the company to work at Abbott Laboratories in Chicago. In addition to that, we lost most of our other marketing people, as well. Most were getting good offers from other companies, but Dick Hearns died of a brain tumor, which was such a tragedy.

Our staffing situation was not our only problem. After the fire in '85, we had to make our products off-site, which increased our production expenses. In addition, we lost a $9 million-dollar contract in South Africa worth 25% of our sales.

Our expansion into Europe and Africa had been a success. While U.S. sales were declining in the 1980s, sales in Africa were increasing. In fact, our products were the leaders in the black hair-care market in both Africa and Britain. Therman had brought in a distributor, Walter Dube, in Lesotho, an enclave in South Africa. Walter was contracted to market and distribute $1.5 million worth of M&M products in South African homelands and nations such as Botswana and Swaziland.

Because South Africa entirely surrounds Lesotho, the small country was inextricably connected with Apartheid, the Afrikaans word for "separation" or "aparthood." It was South Africa's policy of segregation manifest enforced by laws that favored the white minority in power. Apartheid kept non-whites from participating in the national government; they could not vote or hold office. Property was confiscated, and black Africans were prohibited from entering certain areas of the country without permission, which was never granted. They could not run any professional businesses in areas designated "white only."

Lesotho was in constant conflict with South Africa because it supported the African National Congress (ANC), the organization founded in the early 1900s to support and defend the rights of the majority black population. As a black-owned company, Therman and I were proud to have M&M products distributed there. Other companies were in South Africa, such as Alberto and Revlon, but our being in the area had social and political significance. Not only were we a successful black-owned company, but also we supported the boycott of Apartheid and did not do business with South Africa. Because of Lesotho's geographical location, M&M had a face in South Africa, which was positive for black South Africans. We felt like we were saying to them, 'You can make it, too.' The people of South Africa had displayed tremendous dignity under circumstances that could have bent and broken them.

In the late 1980s, however, we were faced with

some difficult choices. Our Lesotho distributor, Walter
Dube, was in the hole to the tune of $250,000.

"Why are we still shipping product to him when he
owes us?" I asked Therman one bright spring day in the
late 1980s. Other than the initial trip to Nigeria with
Therman several years back to set up our initial African
distribution, I had stayed out of this area and focused
my attention on domestic M&M issues. It was beginning to feel like work was a matter of putting out fires
everywhere, not building our business. "He has failed
to sell even half of the amount we contracted with him."

The problem with Walter was that we were send-
ing him hundreds of thousands of dollars worth of
product, but somehow the revenue was not generated.
Some $250,000 later, we were still shipping them.

At the same time, a white-owned, Swaziland-based
company, Vivid U.S. Distributorship Ltd., expressed
interest in taking over distribution. Its president,
Milton Stafford, was impressed with our success in
Nigeria and Lesotho and wanted to bring Sta Sof Fro
and Soft 'n Free products into South Africa.

Like Lesotho, Swaziland is not a part of the
Republic of South Africa, but does share a border with
it. As a result, products would inevitably find their
way into the country that institutionalized racism.
"We should at least meet with them," I told Therman.
"They are willing to come to us."

Therman agreed that we should at least talk to
them. We also agreed that, if we did give Vivid a distributorship, they had to guarantee work in all levels
of the company for local blacks if they did not do so
already, as well as bring in African Americans to work

for the company. "They have got to be integrated," Therman said.

"This is a great opportunity for us to do some good," I continued, thinking of how we could spread our philanthropic activities to a country whose black population was in need of such support. We were both in complete agreement that opportunities at the highest levels should be available to black Africans.

"But we can't leave Walter out," Therman insisted. I grudgingly agreed. Vivid had access to more stores than Walter did, but even though his contract was about to expire, he deserved a chance to work his way out of the money he owed us. Therman, Mack Hunter (M&M's corporate attorney), and I worked out an arrangement that would involve Walter in the Vivid deal.

Before sealing the $9 million contract with Vivid, which gave them the region's sole distribution and marketing rights to M&M products, Mack Hunter and I traveled to South Africa to bring Walter into the deal. "You will no longer be the sole distributor," Mack began, "but you will be a Vivid board member and distributor."

"No!" he shot back in a clipped English accent. "*I* am the distributor for M&M. I asked you for help with marketing. I saw there was a difficulty, and you should help me."

"Walter," Mack interjected, "when you signed the contract, you signed for the marketing of M&M products, too. But you still had access to our departments, and we set up trade shows here. We did support our interests here. It should never have gone this far."

"This is an opportunity," I added calmly, "for you to work your way out of the debt." I shook my head. "It is a sizable one, too."

In the end, a disgruntled Walter agreed to the arrangement. He never acknowledged that he had not lived up to his financial obligations to M&M.

Back in Atlanta, Therman and I met to discuss the South Africa trip. I expressed my dissatisfaction. "I just don't get it. We could demand that money back, but instead, we are keeping him involved."

United in our dealings with Walter, Therman tried to console me. "Come on, man. You and I both know we did the right thing. That's what we've always been about. Even if no one else knows that, *we* know it. It's always been you and me, man. You and me."

For the last time in M&M's history, I felt intensely close to Therman in that moment. It was like old times again, he and I like two peas in a pod. Despite the tension that had been building between Therman and me, one thing was certain: we never stopped trying to make the right decisions. We never stopped trying to do what was right, what would benefit the company, and so also benefit everyone involved. To us, business should be profitable for everyone involved—from the owner to the employee to the customer and everyone in between. It was with this idea in mind that motivated our endeavor with Vivid. Unfortunately, not everyone saw it that way.

In a strange series of events, M&M Products were soon the object of scorn and public speculation about our involvement in South Africa. Everyone had their own opinion about what we were doing, but no one but those of us on the inside of M&M knew the truth. The papers ran with a scandalous story about a black company doing business with South Africa, and, worse yet, drumming out a black African in favor of a business deal with a white company.

It started when we sent Cliff Bowles, M&M's International Division's sales representative, to South Africa to monitor our interests in Lesotho and Swaziland after we completed the Vivid deal. Cliff, who had taken over our international concerns from J. C. Douglas, the man who had started the division for us, happened to run into an old college friend. This friend was now a reporter for the *Atlanta Journal Constitution*. When the reporter learned that Cliff worked for M&M, he started sniffing for a story, and somehow learned about Walter Dube, who he then contacted. Soon thereafter, an article appeared with an incendiary headline accusing M&M of dumping black distributors of M&M products for a white-owned company doing business in the Republic of South Africa. After that, everybody started writing about it.

In mid-June, 1985, I read the *Atlanta Journal Constitution* with my morning coffee, as I usually did. What I read shocked me. In her column, writer Cynthia Tucker claimed that Therman and I "managed to ensnare themselves in a twisted skein of naïveté, miscalculation and poor political judgment." She went on to write that we, "infuriated black businessmen in southern Africa by dumping a black distributor for a white-controlled distribution." Man, I thought to myself. "When you lead and succeed, they call you an entrepreneur. When you lead and fail, they call you naïve."

I picked up the phone and called Therman. "Man, you are not going to believe this." Things had been written about our involvement in South Africa before, and it was based entirely on our disgruntled distributor, Walter Dube.

"It's not true!" a distraught Therman yelled. "How can they print these lies and pass them off for facts?"

"It does not matter if it's true or not. We are already passed that point. What matters now is what people think. They have made a perception game, a public relations exercise." I sighed and shook my head, suddenly thrust back to every experience in which I could not control what was going on—at least not directly. Once people get it into their heads that they know the truth, especially when that truth makes them feel a certain way, it is almost impossible to change their minds. There was no doubt in my mind that this was what was happening with the unfolding South Africa disaster. No matter how much we ranted and raved, it wouldn't matter. The worst part of it was that people were going to help bring down a black-owned company for something that we did not even do. Tucker called us naïve, but it was people like her who were the naïve ones, letting half-truths run off down the road at full speed.

People felt strongly, and rightfully so, about how terrible Apartheid was. So even if it was not true that we were selling our products in the Republic of South Africa, just the hint of it being true was enough to make many people angry.

We tried to respond in the press, explaining both our business connections in the area, as well as our position on Apartheid and our community involvement at home. We explained that we believed substantial black distributorship was in place at Vivid, and pointed out that the company had black executives. We also explained that, if there were no substantial black presence at Vivid, we would sever our ties with that company. We hoped our record would be noticed, and that the truth would come out. It didn't. All anyone knew was that Walter Dube was black, had lost his distributorship, and worst of all, lost it to a white-owned company. He believed that he laid the groundwork for the enormous success Vivid was now enjoying as distributor. In the year since Vivid took over, sales doubled. Depending on how you looked at it, either Walter was right, or the move to Vivid was right because it resulted in a tremendous sales increase.

Soon, Georgia politicians and religious leaders were involved. Though the Rev. Joseph Lowery, of the Southern Christian Leadership Conference (SCLC), agreed that M&M should confirm the presence of black employees at Vivid. But State Rep. Tyrone Brooks asserted that black involvement in Vivid was not relevant, since, "M&M is allowing its products to be sold in South Africa."

We were also taking heat from South Africa's business community. A consultant and former advertising executive, Eric Mafuna, told the *Constitution* that we did not realize "the politics of the situation." What Mr. Mafuna did not realize was that a big part of our business that year was supposed to come from Lesotho and Swaziland, and if we did not have a deal with Vivid, we had nothing else to fall back on, and would lose $9 million. Everyone seemed to have ignored the fact that Walter Dube had been extended $250,000 in credit, and hadn't paid it back.

Perhaps if our products were not so popular in the region, the situation might not have gotten so out of hand. Perhaps if we were not a black-owned company, no one would be concerned. After all, who was asking about Revlon or Alberta, who *were* selling in South Africa? In any case, we were accused of hurting local black businesses in Africa, starting with Walter Dube.

I turned to Coretta Scott King and Andy Young, Atlanta's mayor. Andy had participated in a news conference and publicity event when we signed the initial distribution deal with Walter in the fall of 1983.

"You know who we are," I told Andy. Both Therman and I were close to Andy—Therman particularly so since he became involved in Atlanta's political scene. "And now we are all over CNN!"

Therman could barely contain his emotion. "It's like they just forgot who we are. We co-sponsored the Arthur Ashe event, long before any of this stuff came out, and now they want to say we're some sort of shameful, black-hating company?" Arthur Ashe had sponsored an event which kicked off the movement against apartheid in South Africa, and M&M had donated $25,000. We were involved in the movement almost from the beginning, but no one seemed to notice that significant detail.

The very people who had come to us with their hands out before were now threatening to mount boycotts of all M&M products. Sometimes they even did both at the same time. Therman and I met with a number of local politicians and religious leaders who suggested to us that "donations" might assuage the desire to boycott M&M.

"We cannot pay anyone off just to avoid a boycott, local or nationwide," I said, as Andy listened to our woes. "That's bribery. Besides, we have done nothing wrong. Nothing."

"We have to do what we have to do to stay afloat," Therman countered.

No one wanted to stick his neck out to support us. We were cut loose from almost all of our ties. There were private commiserations, but no public declarations that M&M was getting a raw deal. Andy Young and Maynard Jackson advised us to get out of the South Africa deal as gracefully as possible. There was, they said, no other way to diffuse the conflagration. I traveled to Chicago to seek out advice from Jesse Jackson about avoiding a boycott, but in the end, Therman came up with some money.

I knew Jesse from M&M's support of his P.U.S.H. Coalition, and he received me when I sought a meeting with him. But I knew almost from the moment we shook hands that he did not want to go out for us. It was too much of a political risk. Instead, he referred me to Randall Robinson, who was the president of Trans Africa, the Washington, DC, foreign policy organization. I was disappointed and frustrated since I did not have time to fly all over the country looking for leaders to support M&M.

Finally, M&M severed ties with Vivid, a move we

announced publicly. As a result, M&M products would, at least for the time being, not be available in South Africa. We had lost 25 % of our sales, or what amounted to $9 million. Once we were officially disconnected from the South Africa fiasco, people came forward to endorse us, such as Andy Young and Michael Lomax, Fulton County Commission Chairman. But it was too late. Perception, in this case, was everything, and the result of that perception was financially devastating to M&M.

We tried to rebound by introducing an at-home kit in the Soft 'n Free line. Soft 'n Free Salon Strength no-lye conditioning relaxer system did well in our Atlanta test market, and we expected it to be a big seller nationally.

Still, the effect of the South Africa incident on M&M Products Company was devastating. Sales continued to decline, and we had to cut back even further, eliminating more and more jobs. In this round of cuts, I had to make one of the hardest decisions of my career. I had to let go a long and trusted friend, Eugene Brooks. Brooks was with us from the beginning and contributed to M&M's early development. It was like cutting off one of my arms, and when I told him, I cried. He had come on board early on as a distributor in Memphis, and we were close.

Chapter 19: The Passing of Life, The End Drawing Near

Without a doubt, worse than anything going on in my career was what was happening at home. Sheila's kidneys continued leaking protein and her health continued to deteriorate. She was losing her kidneys. It was time to start thinking about a kidney transplant, and Harriet and I discussed which of us should donate one of our kidneys to our eldest daughter.

I decided I should be the one to do it. Harriet had carried four children, and already had surgeries when she delivered our children by caesarian section. The kidney donation was our last chance to help Sheila, and we were optimistic it would work. Still that time of uncertainty, in both my professional and personal lives, was stressful. I worked to compartmentalize each area of my life so that I could find it endurable, but the stress resulted in a case of hypertension. I kept exercising, continuing the devotion I had begun years ago while in the Air Force, and though it kept me in overall good health, I had difficulty relaxing.

"I see you have to have another drink of wine," Harriet commented, eyebrows arched, one night after dinner.

"I just need to relax," I responded. It seemed I needed a glass every night to relax.

Harriet did not say anything else.

My mother and father were worried enough about my decision to donate a kidney to come see me in the hospital before the operation, hoping to change my mind.

"This is my daughter, my baby," I said to them as they sat by my hospital bed. "I have to do whatever it takes. Whatever it takes."

Sheila responded well at first to the kidney transplant, for about six months. I was relieved I could do something for her. It did not matter what happened to me. I just wanted to help my daughter.

A few months later, my father, however, was not faring as well.

"Cornell." It was my mother's voice on the other end of the telephone line. "Your father's health is failing. You should come on down."

The gaunt figure in my parents' bed looked vaguely like my father. His health had deteriorated severely and rapidly, his body ravaged by the cancer, and now he was in bed, looking small amidst the expanse of bedding that covered him.

I moved to his side and held his hand. His breath was shallow and weak. Patting his hand, I said, "You have that garden looking good, Dad." After sitting with him for a while, I went to make my mother some coffee. When I returned, she was sitting beside him. Light streamed in from across the room, falling gently across my father.

Standing in the doorway, watching them together, my father suddenly reached out his hand, grasping for his wife. "I'm doing all I can," she said gently, taking his hand in hers. "I'm doing all I can."

My father died in 1988. The McBride children coalesced around our mother, caring for her every day. We arranged a calendar rotation so that one of us would be there for her all the time. She had begun to forget her own medications, and having us around kept her steady. I would rotate mostly on the weekends, so that I could be in Atlanta for my family and M&M. There was little time for private grieving, however, because M&M suffered more losses, and we were struggling to save our failing company. Then another fire broke out, disrupting manufacturing once again. Sales continued to slide.

At the same time, Sheila's health began to deteriorate once again. She was not taking care of herself after the operation, and missed a number of follow-up appointments with her doctor. Soon thereafter, her body began to reject my kidney. Upon returning from a trip to South Africa, Harriet and I found a very ill daughter.

"I feel *fine*, overall," I overheard Sheila say to Harriet. "It's just a flu." With medication, a strict diet and close monitoring, Sheila had managed fairly well. But being young, she thought feeling well meant she was well. Though she had been warned that flu-like symptoms were signs of rejection, she had ignored them.

"What's this?" I asked, entering the kitchen.

Sheila turned to me in frustration. "It's nothing, Dad."

"Doesn't sound like nothing." I looked at her a minute, then sighed. She just wanted to be free. Instead, her life was dictated by how she felt from one day to the next, dictated by doctors and the fear that her new kidney would fail. All she wanted was a regular life, and even if she had to deceive herself into it, Sheila was determined to make it happen. "You've stopped taking your medication?"

"I take so many medications, Dad. I'm tired of it."

"Your body will be worse off than tired if you quit your medications. You might feel okay now, but that won't last."

Harriet turned on her heel, saying, "I'm going to call the doctor."

"Mom!" Sheila protested. "I can take care of myself. I'm not a baby."

"Then why don't you act like it!" Harriet snapped. She had endured so much with Sheila, and the prospect of her daughter being ill again and possibly losing her kidney, was too much to bear.

Though I was pained to see what was happening, and unhappy that Sheila had chosen not to do everything she could to be healthy after the transplant, I could not blame her for wanting to put it behind her and finally have a chance at a life. She was 25 years old, but never had the opportunity to enjoy her youth or blossom into womanhood.

When we got to the doctor's office, the news was not good. The kidney was lost. "Remember we talked about rejection," the doctor told Sheila. "Your body did not accept your father's kidney, and now it's not working." Her other kidney was already non-functional. "We'll need to start you on dialysis right away."

Sheila started crying, and Harriet tried to comfort her. "I don't want to do this anymore," Sheila sobbed. "I am tired of doctors and hospitals. I am tired of treatments. I just want a normal life."

Sheila lost her kidney, and had to begin dialysis. Her doctor sent her home with a dialysis machine so she would not have to frequent the hospital so much, but her health continued to decline, just as M&M's health did.

M&M Products Company was once the 11th-ranked black-owned company in the nation, according to *Black Enterprise* magazine. By 1989, after struggling in the curl market, and surviving the South Africa debacle, we had dropped to 36th, with less than 200 employees.

Money was lost not just in the domestic market and through the South Africa debacle, but also through deals that collapsed. A good friend of mine, Comer Cottrel, from Proline Corporation in Dallas, Texas, had made an offer to buy M&M's Plastics Division. We made our own bottles for all our products, and Comer wanted to buy it. He offered a million dollars, which Therman and I agreed was a much-needed cash infusion for the company. We decided to add $800,000 of our own retirement money to help keep M&M afloat. At the last minute, however, just as he was about to fly

out to Atlanta to sign the deal, Comer backed out of
the deal. Even though we had a friendship and a verbal agreement, he contended that it wasn't worth it.
Desperate not to lose the deal, I tried to negotiate a
lower offer, but the deal was dead, and we were out
$800,000 of our own retirement money.

As M&M lost money, the banks required us to
bring in "Turnaround Specialists" Coopers & Lybrand
to help us turn M&M around. But at $50,000 a month
in consulting fees, we were being bled dry. How they
expected us to recoup our company under those con-
ditions was anyone's guess. Around Christmas time,
the consultants told us to sell the company. That day, I
drove home with tears streaming down my face. After
all I had done, I felt like a complete failure. This was
one of the lowest points of my life.

Therman seemed to take the recommendation in
stride. He had started a minority consulting firm with
help of his political connections, and he was happy to
move on. "We can go our separate ways," he told me.
I did not want that. Instead, I turned my attention to
making deals that could save M&M.

I was working on a proposal to sell the
International Distribution deal to AMKA Cosmetics
when Laf came to me. "I got a call from Bert Lee. He is
interested in buying M&M, and I think it could work.
You know things aren't getting any better the way they
are now," he said, alluding to everything that had happened up to this point. Bertram M. Lee owned BML
Associates Inc., a Boston-based, black-owned firm.

I went to Therman to inform him of Bert's interest, and he practically jumped on it. "Let's do it. Let's
get out now."

I was stunned. Somehow, I refused to believe Therman really wanted out of our company. "You can't—are you serious?"

"Yes," he said flatly. "I am tired of this. Aren't you?"

I still believed we could pull M&M out of its slump. "Therman, this is ours. *Ours.* Why do you want to give it up?"

"I told you, man. Enough is enough."

"Therman, listen. We have to stay strong. I know it has been tough, believe me. But we cannot give up now." I was not thinking just of our business, but the responsibility I felt we had to stay in the industry. Though started by black entrepreneurs such as George Johnson, the "ethnic" hair-care, white-owned companies increasingly dominated the lucrative market.

Not only that, I wanted to prove to everyone that we could rebound and rebuild to meet and exceed our previous financial standing. We had been accused in the press of failing to adjust quickly enough to the curl market, and not planning at all to develop products for later styles, and though this was partly true, it was not the whole truth. We had made mistakes, there was no doubt, but they were always mistakes made in an effort to do right by our company, vendors, employees and customers.

"There could still be a role for us," Therman offered. Maybe he was moved by my plea. "But we need the sort of backing BML could give us."

"They won't be giving us anything," I countered. "They will *own* us." I paused for a moment to look at my good friend, wondering what had happened to us.

Therman had made his decision, and there was nothing else I could do. We informed our employees of our decision, telling them that it was a tough one to make, but that the deal would make M&M secure in a way it currently was not.

I drove home that night, a wave of emotion washing over me. I had not felt like a failure in years, but I did that night, and it sat like a heavy weight in the pit of my stomach. I went from being successful, secure and respected, to feeling almost entirely worthless.

And so the negotiation process started. Bert put Ron Wilburn on to manage the acquisition talks for him, and Mack Hunter, our general counsel, negotiated our part. The mood at M&M deteriorated, despite Therman's and my attempts at smoothing over everyone's concerns. Departments went into panic mode, everyone worrying that their jobs would be the next to go. In a way, we all had people in the company we were trying to protect. Every time I had to look at another list of jobs to cut, I felt utterly drained.

Negotiations with BML dragged on—too long. Since Therman and I had no previous experience selling a company, we had to go along with the buyer. Besides that, Lee was committed to keeping M&M in Atlanta, which meant our employees' job security would not be compromised. But as the process lagged, Laf began to have suspicions that Bert did not have the money to close the deal, and I agreed. When I shared those concerns with Therman, however, he was not willing to walk away.

"Therman, we have got to close this deal. This limbo is not good for any of us," I said in July of 1989.

We had been in negotiations since April. "Besides, AMKA wants to buy the European rights, and that deal is stalled while we sit on our hands and wait on Bert. We need that money."

"Well, why don't you take that up with Laf?" he answered derisively. "He's your dealmaker."

"Don't say that, man, this was your idea. This is all you. I never wanted to sell."

"It will happen. Just give it time."

"Time is what we do not have. We have a deadline, and if he does not make it, the deal is off."

I left Therman's office in frustration, and tracked Lafayette Jones down. "I'm going to call Bert myself," I said. As a member of the First America Bank board, I put feelers out to find out what was keeping Bert from closing the deal. It was a good deal for him, too. In fact, it favored his financial interests more than ours, since it gave him five years to pay for the company, which would be five years the McKenzie and McBride families would not see any money. With Therman and I practically financing the deal, I could not figure out what the hold-up was. What I learned from my bank contacts was that Lee was shopping around for the money. I was infuriated to learn that he did not have the capital to come up with even the minimum amount to close a deal that would give him five years to pay off the bulk!

Laf gave me Bert's number, and I called him at home that Sunday. "Why are you calling me at home?" Bert said, annoyed. "And on a Sunday."

"We need to talk."

"Can't it wait until Monday?"

"No, it cannot. We have waited long enough already." There was silence on the end of the line, so I continued. "We have already gone through two closing dates. There is another one coming up, and this one has to be met." Still, there was silence. "Mr. Lee, if you do not close by the next deadline, I will have to go talk to someone else."

Finally, he responded. "I will close when I get good and ready."

The conversation was over, and I immediately called Therman, Laf, our attorney and other executives. "He does not have the money," I said. "The deal is not going to happen. We have got to call AMKA."

Representatives of the Kalla family of AMKA Cosmetics were in Atlanta, check in hand, the following week. Once Therman saw the check, he was happy to drop the Bert Lee deal and search for another. The infusion of $1 million dollars to secure distribution rights in Europe and Africa was a godsend for us, but it would not save the company in the end.

By July of 1989, I decided I would try to buy M&M. I went to Laf and he agreed to come on board. We also involved John Henderson, a finance guy Lee had brought in when we were negotiating that deal. But when I went to Therman with my offer, he would have none of it.

"If I'm selling, I want my money now," he said flatly.

"Why? You were going to give Bert Lee five *years* to give you money. I just want to save what we started."

But Therman would hear none of it, and his

demand for cash up front made raising money impossible. At one point, Laf, John and I flew to California to see if we could raise some capital through Mike Milkin, the Drexel Burnham Lambert financial executive later called "the junk bond king." We could not get money there, either, though I suspected it was because Milkin was in bed with Johnson Products, which wanted to buy M&M.

Finally, when I had just about exhausted all my options, I called George Johnson. I told him that if I could not raise the money to buy out Therman, I would sell to George. Almost immediately, Therman hired lawyers to try to force me to sell to George Johnson. Meetings were arranged, and I would simply leave the building. I was not about to be forced into anything. Needless to say, Therman and I did not talk too much during those last summer months of M&M's existence.

In October of 1989, I gave up my quest to buy M&M Products, and turned to George Johnson. Chicago's Johnson Products Company offered $5.2 million for all four of our brands, the original Sta Sof Fro, Soft 'n Free, our economy brand Moxie, and Curly Perm, which was created by Therman. Johnson bought the intellectual properties, not anything else– not the plants, etc. They essentially brought the brands and inventory into their own existing company production. Selling Sta Sof Fro felt like selling a child. "Once the deal goes through in February," Therman declared, "I'm moving on."

Somehow I believed that, even if we sold M&M

Products, we could somehow salvage our relationship. After all, we were friends who had accomplished so much together, and I thought we could be friends again. But he was ready to move on.

"I've got other things I want to pursue," he simply said. "There is nothing left for me here."

Though emotionally devastating at the time, it turned out to be a good thing, because I would start over with a clean slate. On February 1, 1990 Therman and I signed the papers to sell M&M Products to Johnson Products. It was one of the lowest points in my life.

At the time, I had a glimmer of hope that I could still run M&M. Though Therman wanted no part of it, I signed on to run M&M as a division of Johnson Products. In February, just after the deal was signed, I flew out to California to meet Eric Johnson, George Johnson's son, where he was attending a series of hair shows in Orange County and San Diego. He and I planned to hammer out the details of M&M's future, which was already put in place before the company was sold. But as I left for California, Harriet's wise voice warned me off this new path.

"Why are you doing this?" she asked. "You know you won't be able to work with them."

"No, it will be fine," I said. I was relieved that Johnson Products was a black-owned company, and that I would have a crucial role to play in the future of M&M. It wasn't fine. Needless to say, Harriet was right.

Eric, it turned out, was a tyrant. His people were scared to death of him, and the atmosphere was asphyxiating. It took me two days to realize that I had the title of Division Head in name only. Eric was making all the decisions—many of which were contrary to what had been agreed to before the company was sold. Specifically, Eric had decided to remove our "green" line, which was under the Soft 'n Free brand, from select distribution. He wanted to sell it to whoever wanted it, and I was adamantly opposed to that idea. But when I tried to discuss it with him, he cut me off.

Finally, I'd had enough. As Eric and I stood in a booth at the San Diego show, surrounded by Johnson employees and hundreds of vendors and stylists, I let loose. "I do not need this!" I practically shouted. "I don't know who you think you are, but I am not having any of it. I've got someplace else to be." With that, I severed my relationship with Johnson Products.

That someplace else was my own company. I would start over with an entirely clean slate. When negotiating the deal to sell M&M, I had made sure the noncompete agreement was taken out. Though standard in sales such as the one between M&M and Johnson, the noncompete agreement kept the seller from starting another company for five years after the sale. Since I was not subject to such a restriction, I gathered my family around, and decided to form a new company, one that would manifest all the ideals and principles I had learned and worked to achieve my entire life. Though the loss of M&M had been heartbreaking, this new beginning was looking more and more like a blessing.

I brought some former employees with me to begin R&D, and though many said I should stop and take a break, that was unthinkable to me. Looking back, however, part of my motivation was to keep moving. If I stopped, I feared the grief over my father's death, and the intense deterioration of my daughter's health would overtake me.

As Sheila became weaker and weaker, we tried to make it as normal as possible, but things had been far from normal for some time. Sheila was in and out of the hospital despite home dialysis, until one day she did not come home. Sheila McBride died of kidney failure in December 1990.

After she died, we received more stunning news. The coroner put the cause of death as AIDS. Confused and angry, I raced to her doctor's office. Had she contracted the disease during her many transfusions in the early '80s? At the time, there was enormous social stigma attached to the disease, and so little was known about it, that it seemed like my baby was suffering all over again.

Her doctor assured me that Sheila did not have AIDS, yet her symptoms were so similar. She had tuberculosis, the fevers, all of it, and she had become so small, so frail that I ached just looking at her. In the end, the worst part was watching her waste away like she did, so gradually and so painfully. Our family will never know for sure exactly how Sheila died, all we know is that she is no longer with us, where she belongs.

Chapter 20: From Out of the Ashes, McBride Research Laboratories

Children, no matter what age, are not supposed to die before their parents. Harriet and I moved quietly around our house, clinging to each other and our remaining children, Cornell Jr., Sholanda and André. Thoughts of Sheila flooded every waking moment, and also my dreams. "I could not save her, I could not save her, I could not save her," looped endlessly in my mind. I kept asking myself what I could have done differently, or more, or less. What choice had I made that led to the way life was now?

We are the products of our own decisions. Bad decisions ripple through our lives with lasting consequences. Good ones do, too, but most often we do not relive everything that led up to the moment the good decision was made. With the bad ones, on the other hand, it is easy to live in a purgatory of regret. I knew I had to decide not to live that life. I could not prevent Sheila from dying, but I could donate a kidney. I could not prevent my father from dying, but I could provide the best doctors and work to alleviate stress for both of my parents, and I could go home to visit often. I could not change the relationship I had with Therman—it was destroyed—but I could find a way to make the transition of selling M&M Products Company as smooth as possible for everyone involved.

Still, I could not help feeling that the failure of M&M was somehow an indictment on me, a reflection of my worth as a person. Within two years I had lost my father, my company and then my daughter. With Sheila's death, I was at my lowest. I remember someone said of me once that I was so optimistic, if I fell off a tall building, as I passed the fourth and then third and then second floors, "Well, at least I haven't hit the ground, yet." But there I was, flat out on the pavement.

Compartmentalizing things happening in my life were taking their toll, and I was tired. I took every excuse to drink wine. It's raining, I'll have a drink of white wine. I'm tired, I'll have a drink of red wine. But, when I woke up, I was still tired.

After Sheila died, I looked around and saw my family. My beautiful and loyal wife, who had stood by me since we were kids, and who had given me four extraordinary children, was still there next to me. My children were all part of my new business. I had safety and security. I had all the love they could give me, and that was all I needed. I decided to stop drinking, and once the decision was made, that was that. I quit, cold turkey. Though later I would have an occasional drink, I replaced the nighttime sleep aid with news tapes. I subscribed to News Track, a service that sends tapes of news summaries, and also bought books on tape, such as history and religion series. Every night, instead of a glass of wine, I dropped a tape in a cassette player and listened until I drifted off to sleep. I was not an alcoholic, but I had been slowly losing control. Fortunately for me, my ability to foresee future trends applied in my personal life. I knew I needed to take charge before I started having a problem with alcohol.

There are things that are outside of our control, and learning what those things are may take years of studying one's own life. But once you learn what you can do and what you can't do, you must pursue what you can do, and accept what you cannot. A large part of taking risks and becoming a success depends on knowing this difference.

With the support of my family, I reoriented my life and focused on building my new company. Though I did it because I wanted to, there were financial reasons motivating me, too.

Immediately after the sale of M&M, I had to consider my financial situation. I had a lot of personal assets, but when M&M left, so did my cash. Within two years of selling M&M, I sold off the remaining Jolly Mack and White's Discount Beauty Supply stores to cut further losses there and to generate some cash. Though I sold assets and reduced expenses, I had created a lifestyle for myself and my family that required cash to maintain, and I knew already that I would start another business, and that required capital.

"McBride Research Laboratories," I told my family one night as we ate dinner. "I know this industry, I was successful in it, and I'm going to be a success again."

"But what if it does not work out?" Harriet asked.

She knew that, despite my experience and success in the hair-care industry, it was hard to make a new start.

"I have to take that chance," I responded.

Cornell Jr. said, "Well, you'd better be ready to take me along."

I smiled. "Come on then. We have a lot of work to do!"

A lot of work was an understatement. With the money I had, I was able to get the new business off the ground. At the end of two years, McBride Research Laboratories was closing in on $1.2 million in sales, and my entire family was working on this new venture with me.

Things were going well, but as with M&M, I needed more capital—I figured about $250,000—to get to the next level. I also knew, from my time on bank boards, that loan applications are thoroughly scrutinized even before they come before a board for a final decision. Loan officers won't originate a loan unless they think it is going to go through. Given my background, I believed there would be no problem finding the additional funding I needed for McBride Research Laboratories.

I learned quickly, however, that my proven track record meant nothing to the big banks, which is where I went initially. I needed about $300,000, and believed the larger banks, with which M&M had done business, were the places to go. There was a minority loan program through the NAACP, and I went to Citizens and National Bank (later Nations Bank) to fill out the application. After a month, when I heard nothing from them, I went back.

"The head office turned you down," the loan officer said.

"Nobody was going to bother to tell me?" I asked.

"I'm sorry," he shrugged noncommittally.

"Look, if you don't trust that I can execute the plan I submitted to you, why don't you stage perform the loan?" Stage performance meant giving a portion of the loan, and then, based on performance, giving out the rest. I did not need all of the money at once, and could have gotten started with a fraction.

At that point, the loan officer got frustrated. I did not simply go away when denied, but instead had offered an alternative. "I can't help you," he answered snidely.

"What is it, man? I never even got an interview. That's standard. No one ever came to my business. Again, standard. I'm already going into my third year—"

He cut me off. Jabbing a finger at me, he said, "You need to go where somebody knows you."

"This is a waste of time," I said, and walked out.

Another loan fell through before I found one, literally, next door. Sometimes, good advice can come from unlikely places. I did go where somebody knew me: my next-door neighbor, Gregory Baranco, was the chairman of First Southern Bank, a small, black-owned institution. It had not occurred to me to consider it before because it was such a small bank. But it turned out to be the best decision I made.

"Mr. McBride," Herb Reese greeted me with extended hand. "I'm glad you decided to come to us." Herb was the president of First Southern, and he was eager to make the loan.

Reese was taking a chance on me, there was no doubt about that. Even though the federal government regulated First Southern, just as it did the larger banks, First Southern's asset base was much smaller. So, if I failed, the effect on the bank would be detrimental. A large bank, on the other hand, would not have even felt a bump.

Lending money is not a science, as some people might try to make you think it is. In the end, lending money is about having good reasons to give someone money. Fortunately, Reese saw those good reasons in me. I had a history of success and hard assets to back up the loan.

Later, it seemed to me that the NAACP program was, for a lot of banks, just performing the fashion. The federal government's Community Reinvestment Act (CRA) required that, every quarter as part of their charter, banks had to show that they were loaning money to minorities. The NAACP program was mostly for show. The moment the quota was met, loans stopped going out. Banks even put on seminars to show how helping minorities worked. I never could figure out what the big mystery was about lending money to black people. It was as if we were a different species from everyone else. Business is business, no matter what color you are. What I had learned was that you have to have more just to get a little bit. A successful black man, in the white world of business, was considered something strange. There was a deeper meaning to success for a black person, a lack of respect for success achieved, as if, instead of being smart and hardworking, the person was just lucky.

Now, almost 15 years later, McBride Research Laboratories is a multimillion-dollar company, with a distribution model that has helped our people earn six-figure incomes year after year. We also have a complete distribution business whose success rivals the dominant supply chains, such as Sally's.

Everything that I had wanted to do with M&M Products Company I am doing now with McBride Research Laboratories. I have learned from both my mistakes and my successes, and this knowledge has been poured, down to the last drop, into my company. The business model that focuses on making money for both the company and the company's distributor means that we're in this thing together. If I win, they win; if they win, I win. I have always believed that businesses are community ventures. A business touches everyone in the community in some way, and as far as I am concerned, my business has a responsibility to keep that relationship healthy. With this approach, I avoid problems such as the South Africa incident that led to the downfall of M&M.

Everyone affiliated with McBride Research Laboratories goes through a continual educational process so that he or she can learn about the fiscal discipline that helped create my success. I travel the country talking to people who are struggling to make it, but often do not have the know-how to do it. "Free your mind," I tell them. "If your mind is free from distraction, that means it's free to learn something new, to have time to think about how you can be *creative* and make more for yourself."

Especially today, with so many people toiling away

but finding themselves deeper and deeper in debt, a free mind is hard to find. People are preoccupied with how to just make that next bill payment, preoccupied with just trying to catch up, that they never get ahead. "If the money on the dresser does not belong to you, I say (recalling the time I put cash that belonged to M&M on my bedroom dresser and refused to use any of it for my personal purposes), don't use it. Whenever there is a struggle, it's tempting to give in to it, to just give up. But you have got to stay strong and be disciplined."

Thirty years ago, M&M Products left the basement of my home and went on to become a multimillion-dollar international concern. Now, here I am once again, working every day to make the right decisions for my company, my employees, distributors, clients and everyone whose lives are affected by McBride Research Laboratories and its products, Design Essentials and Wave by Design. By sticking to lifelong principles, everything has come full circle. I did not get it right all the time, but I stayed with it, corrected my mistakes and kept looking to the future. All the challenges and difficulties I faced throughout my life were never insurmountable because I lived by the Godly principles learned on Mom's table when I was a little boy growing in Savannah, Georgia. The values of fairness, honesty, hard work, discipline she taught me never left me all these years. They are the solid foundation of my life and that of my family. We never waver in our trust in God's grace and goodness. How great to know that God is good.

Epilogue

People always ask me how I did it. They want to know how I became a multi-millionaire, not once, but twice. They want to know how I built two successful companies from the ground up. It's as if they think I had some magic formula, some secret to success, and if they could just get their hands on it, they'd become financially successful, too. For a long time I thought about it, wondering what it was that made my professional life different from so many others. At times, the question was like a terrible pressure to come up with a brilliant, completely original idea that, when applied to life, quickly and easily moves one into prosperity. And then it hit me. The idea is brilliant, but it's not original to me. Many people aren't going to like it, because it's not going to give them an easy route to riches. But neither of those things matter because it's an idea that anyone can apply in life, and it works.

What's my secret to success? Valuing honesty, hard work, determination, discipline, creativity, and family. You can't have a shortcut to those types of value. They take time to develop. I was fortunate enough to be born with a knack for recognizing a good thing when I see it. But, by itself, that's not enough. You have to be able to know what to do with that good thing, or, if you don't know, be creative enough to find out what you can do. Creativity requires hard work, discipline, and determination. If we all waited around for inspiration, most ideas would never get off the ground. Hard work develops those ideas through creativity, and, while discipline keeps the hard work going, it is determination that steers you forward to realize your dream. Of course, none of these things has quite as much value as family, but with family by your side, the rewards bestowed by those values are sweet.

So, you see, I have no magic pill for success. I have only the same values that can make any American prosper.